DR LINDA WILSON

STRESS
made easy!

PEELING WOMEN
OFF THE CEILING

With sincere thanks to Rafael Topolski for the cover design and all the other design work you have done. Raf you are an artist. raf.topolski@gmail

To my editor Lisa Cropman, thank you for your gentle pushes and thoughtful insight. I appreciate it. www.thewordnest.com.au

I could not have completed this book with out the wonderful support of my family. Andrew thank you for helping me make my dream come true. Isaac and Isobel your patience over the months I locked myself away was awesome. Thank you family with all my love.

Dedicated in loving memory of my Dad
Ian William Wilson and my Aunty Jennifer Mary Wilson.

National Library of Australia Cataloguing-in-Publication details:

Creator:	Wilson, Linda, author
Title:	Stress made easy: peeling women off the ceiling / Dr Linda Wilson
ISBN:	9780992516550 (paperback)
Subjects:	Stress management for women – Popular works
	Stress management – Popular works
	Stress (Psychology) – Popular works
	Anxiety in women – Popular works
	Women – Health and hygiene – Popular works
Dewey Number:	155.9042

Cover design by Rafael Topolski
Interior design by Michael Hanrahan Publishing
Printed in Australia

Contents

Introduction

All of us have stress, even if we don't admit it. And for some of us, it's crippling.

During my 15 years practicing as a stress specialist, working with and learning from mentors and clients (as well as dealing with my own stress), I've heard these questions many times: 'Why do I feel so stressed?' and 'How can I manage my stress?' This book has been written to answer such questions and to help you understand that reducing your stress is achievable, it's in your power and it's one of the most important things you can do for yourself and those around you.

As you will discover, there have been many times I've had to 'peel myself off the ceiling' as my stress threatened to overwhelm me. I hope my passion to find tools and techniques that actually work makes your journey a less stressed one. I speak from a woman's perspective, however, having seen many male clients over the years, I know that all the tools and techniques easily cross over the gender divide. This book is all about Stress Made Easy – for everyone.

Given that we are the most advanced animal species, (with the interpretation of 'advanced' being debatable), it does seem ridiculous that we spend enormous amounts of our time stressed, anxious, worried, depressed, sad, defeated, angry, resigned, triggered and disappointed.

As you'll read in the pages to follow, a growing body of scientific evidence proves that negative stress and even *thinking* about the negative effects of stress, is damaging our health. So, isn't it about time we learnt how to take responsibility for our wellbeing? For whilst it may seem that there's nothing you can do about stress (there will always be bills, responsibilities, demands and challenges from the past, now in the present and in the future), you have more control than you think. My motto has always been 'change your mind, change our world', and this will make more sense as you move through the chapters.

In the first part of this book, I explain why you feel stress the way you do, so that you learn to recognise how your own stress patterns are created and perpetuated. We explore how the meaning makes all the difference to how you perceive and respond to a trigger and how you have the power to change it.

In the part two, I introduce you to the actual tools and techniques and finally 'ADAPTability', my 5-step process designed to guide you through recognising and transforming the way you hold and process thoughts, react to feelings and perpetuate outdated beliefs. Both parts of the book will help you to understand and respond to stressful situations in positive and practical ways, so you feel calm, confident, connected and in control.

This book is a resource that can be used in a number of ways:

1. You can read the book from start to finish and then come back to the end of each chapter to do each reader activity.

2. You can read the book from start to finish, completing each reader activity as you go.

3. If you're keen to get straight to the tools and techniques and learn about the theory later, you can start at chapter 13, returning to chapters 1–12 to gain more insight into the process.

I use the ADAPTability model (see chapter 16) with all my clients. ADAPTability combines Hypnotherapy, Neuro Linguistic Programming and Cognitive Behavioural Therapy with Traditional Chinese Medicine, Energy Psychology and 'The Quick Tap' practice of Faster

Emotionally Focused Transformations. In short, my technique fuses the best of cutting edge science with ancient wisdoms to address the mind-body system as one. Using the body to inform the mind and vice versa is the only way to be truly congruent with ourselves.

This easy-to-learn, step-by-step process has helped my clients achieve rapid life-changing breakthroughs and sustained results, even in the most challenging circumstances.

So – are you stressed out enough to take a risk on learning something new? Something that may challenge the way you have always viewed yourself and the rest of the world? A risk on happiness? A risk on change? Do you want to achieve rapid and dynamic transformation? This is exactly what's on offer in the pages of this book.

Start changing your life today by using the simple process I reveal. Enjoy the freedom to choose your reactions to stress and escape the effects that, left unchecked, will undermine your physical and emotional health.

Don't miss this opportunity to take a moment to check-in with yourself with positive regard; to create, to connect and to celebrate your incredible ability to experience relaxation, calm, happiness, peacefulness, satisfaction and fulfillment.

Good luck on your journey, and know that you are not alone in your search for a more connected, centred and peaceful you.

Part 1

Insight into Stress

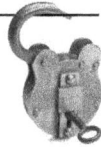

Chapter 1

Why do we feel stress?

What is stress?

We're all born with an instinctive stress response. Triggered when faced with threat or challenge, stress hormones are released into our bloodstream and prepare us to 'freeze', 'fight' or run away, 'flight'. The mental and physical changes stress provokes fill us with stamina, speed and strength. Our stress response has enabled our species to survive.

These days, when we are less likely to be physically threatened, we still experience the same stress response when faced with challenge. It helps us to perform under pressure and keeps us focused, energised and alert. But beyond a certain point, and without sufficient down time, stress stops being helpful and starts causing major damage.

The complexity of modern life has made many of us hooked on stress so that we're on constant alert. We become habituated to our stress levels and the kind of hurried, tense lifestyle that's characteristic of our fast-paced culture. In some instances, we become adrenaline junkies fixated on the next natural chemical high. We can even become bored when we don't have the hormones of stress and excitement humming through our brains and bodies. We take pride in multitasking mastery and find it hard to switch off and relax. Our bodies don't have time to rest after each stress-filled moment and we are perpetually ready to fight or take flight. Long-term exposure to stress can lead to serious health problems – and threaten to sabotage our very survival.

This is more than theory and conjecture. Let's look at some of the numbers associated with stress: In 2013, Safe Work Australia reported that Australian businesses lost more than $10 billion due to work related mental stress[1]. (In 2008, Medicare put the figure above $14 billion.) On its website, Work Safe Australia states that, 'Stress is the second most common cause of compensation claims in Victoria, Australia after manual handling'[2]. Consider the repercussions of these statistics. Consider how our health is suffering.

I believe that one of the problems of the modern age is that we are preoccupied with negative aspects of life. Bad news sells; we are entertained by doom and gloom, drama, danger and death, and all too often the bad is overinflated and the good goes unnoticed. But why are we so fascinated with the negative?

Well, if we set aside simple laziness as the issue, (after all it takes more mental discipline and effort to spend time in a positive frame of mind and environment), what we are left with is what 'grabs' us, what gives us a rush and what is served up to us via the media and entertainment industries. Drama sells.

Many of us don't realise the full effect that stress has on our lives until its too late. To manage stress we need to check in on ourselves with inquisitive and non-judgmental regard. Connecting mind and body is key to this process – as is understanding how the mind creates meaning to stimulate the body's stress response. In my practice, and in this book, my aim is to encourage focused understanding of our stress responses so that we can dismantle the automatic thoughts, feelings and reactions that keep us in our stressed states.

Stress – a conflict between expectations and reality

We have little control over life events but we do have the ability to adapt to them. Most of the time we are able to adapt physically and emotionally to events and situations. But sometimes, when we are unable to adapt it creates internal struggle and this causes stress. Simply put, stress happens when life doesn't go according to our hopes or plans.

Let's look at life as a game. The set of rules with which we are raised is our 'belief system'. Our beliefs shape the way we view every-thing and live and experience life. Our expectations and view of life are then filtered through the lens of our belief system and so on. Through the experiences we have and the meanings we give those experiences, we have an understanding about how things are supposed to operate. This includes us, other people, family, friends, our community, society and the world at large. We view the world through our belief system and have no choice but to filter everything we see, feel, hear, taste and touch through what *already* exists within us. This means *everything* is distorted because it is coming via an 'already expecting' framework. Is this bad? Is this good? It's neither. It just *is*.

We develop values, morals, anticipations and expectations in an ever-expanding collection of experiences that affirm or offend our beliefs. When we see something that fits within our expectations and beliefs about the world, we gravitate towards it and it affirms our belief system. We believe we are right to see the world in this way – it is *so*. When we see something that doesn't fit within our existing framework of expectations and beliefs, we naturally ques-tion it. It may not affirm our knowledge of the world or our under-standing of ourselves – so how can it possibly be *so*?

When reality and expectation don't align

In the instances when we are challenged by an experience that 'doesn't fit' with our rules or expectations, two things can happen:

1. We respond with positive curiosity and a desire to know more. The mind's job is to find a way to absorb newness into our *known* understanding of the world. However, with curiosity we can learn new ways of seeing and experiencing our world that may produce wonderful opportunities for personal development and provide enriching and fulfilling chapters in our life.

2. Because the mind's job is to find a way to absorb newness into our *known* understanding of the world, challenging experiences can also produce negative feelings including stress, fear and anger. The entire array of hurtful, harmful and negative feelings can be generated via this new experience in the same way as the whole array of wonderful, enriching and fulfilling experiences can too.

All perspectives are overlaid and interpreted through the meaning we give them based on our expectations and beliefs about how our world fits together – our *'this is so'* and how rigid and inflexible we are in our point of view. To a certain extent we are incapable of absorbing new experiences without challenging our beliefs.

To illustrate the point, here are some simple examples of how stress is generated by differences in expectations and beliefs:

You set out a work project into incremental timeframes. Your colleague prefers to go with the flow. He takes this to mean you are uptight. You take this to mean he's lazy. Your beliefs about how the project *should* be handled are different. This causes stress.

You believe the toothpaste lid should be put back after each use. Your partner doesn't see this as important. You see your partner as slovenly. Your partner sees you as neurotic. These differences in expectation create stress.

Wherever there is difference, there is opportunity. We choose the meaning of every experience and this determines how we feel about it – good, bad or indifferent.

The opportunity to experience difference comes up all the time as we interact with others and their different rules of the game. Our expectations and beliefs about the world and our relationships are challenged in every moment as we *expect* and *believe* our way through the day. We can choose how it impacts us by using this awareness as a guide. We can choose whether to see these challenges as positive, negative or just plain different. We can choose to interpret these experiences through the eyes of stressed positive curiosity or stressed negative challenge.

Another way of explaining negative stress is as a result of the oppositional ways individuals live by the rules of their game. We can choose to be right and offended by others and their view of the world (righteous) or we can choose to be curious and see every difference as an opportunity to learn about different rules.

Can you change your beliefs and expectations in order to reduce your experience of stress? Yes you can, but only if you want to. The insights you'll find in the pages of this book will help you do just that.

Reader Activity

- Consider where you spend your time and with whom. What does this provoke in you?

- Do a quick assessment of the percentage of time you spend risk assessing, averting, managing or analysing. Most importantly, when you go within, what percentage of time are you dealing with the same stressors?

- Do you anticipate the worst, expect a poor result and resign yourself to inevitable disappointment?

- Are your stress levels linked to this preoccupation with the negative?

- Does your stress 'stress you out'?

- Does it add or subtract from the quality of your day, your relationships, your work?

Summary

- We are just as capable of being happy as we are of being stressed.

- Stress is a lazy response because it doesn't require consciousness and evaluation.

- Happiness requires an active choice.

- Remaining curious about our reactions can help us change them.

- The good news is you can get to choose.

NOTES

NOTES

Chapter 2

The game of life is set up with inherited rules

When we play a game of chess, Monopoly or any board game there is always a 'set up' required. In my house, my youngest child takes great pride in making sure all the bits and pieces of the game are set up and everyone has exactly what they need.

The interesting thing about this is that life is the same. We often think our life or our 'emotional story' begins from the moment we are born, but in many ways we are already designed before we even appear – 'who we are' and 'how we are' is already set up and ready to go. We are a blank canvas yet there has been a huge number of moves already made and stories created before we even arrive.

The set up

So, how are we set up to play our game in a real life situation?

Well, you began with two people who contributed a part of themselves that became you. They may not have been aware at the time that you were going to be the result. They may not have been the people that ultimately raised you – but someone did, either by their presence or by their absence. If you had parents or people around you who were capable of nourishing and caring for a child you were lucky. If they weren't capable, you were not. The point is, whoever raised you had their problems and beliefs. They bought with them all the ways they believed life should be set up, their own set of rules, their own cheat sheet, their own idea of who else should be playing the game with them and how. All that information was already there before you were conceived.

Inheriting beliefs, problems, expectations

You enter the scene at the moment of your birth. All of the circum-stances surrounding your birth, all of the people involved in your creation and all of their beliefs, problems and expectations are right there ready to be written into your rule book. This is an inheritance you can't escape. Can you see that so many moves had already been made before you even entered the game room?

The people who raise you teach you the rules of their game, as they know them. What else can they do but teach you their version of the rules? They have nothing else to go on except the way they have always known it to be, the way they have always played. The rules you are taught are the best version they are capable of coming up with according to their history. The rules are their beliefs, problems and expectations both for you and about you.

You learn these rules well because you know if you don't play by the rules you won't fit in.

Creating an identity according to the rules

From the rules you are taught you became very clear about who you are and who you're not. For example, you are a 'quiet', 'good' and 'invisible' person' or a 'funny', 'helpful' and 'creative' person. You learn about where you fit and where you don't, and why this is so. You learn how to be a good player according to the family rules. You learn just as much from the omissions in the rulebook as what's written down in black and white and spoken of clearly. You become who you are within your family game and then you extend that out into the wider community.

Interacting with others using this identity

Wherever you are, you take your identity with you. When you begin to spread your wings, it's usually amongst a small circle of friends and family. Your identity is affirmed because you are playing by their rules. You are recognised and accepted amongst this group. You start to truly believe you are who they say you are. You strengthen your belief that 'this is who I am' and 'this is how the game is played'. You go out into the world and start practicing 'being' your identity, out there amongst the other players.

Finding people who sit well with your identity (because they make you feel OK)

This is a good place to introduce you to the concept of your brain's Reticular Activating System or RAS. Put simply, this is the system through which nearly all information enters the brain (smells are the exception; they go directly to the brain's emotional area). The RAS filters incoming information and focuses attention. Its job is to find what you are looking for and disregard all else.

Your RAS recognises things that are important to your survival. When I was little, I always walked with my head down looking at the ground. I did this because I grew up in the desert and we had to be careful of snakes. It was important to my survival that I find any snakes that were on my path. A number of times I actually did. A number of times I believed long sticks, bits of rubber, wire, vines and various other bits of rubbish were snakes as well because my mind would turn these things into what I was looking for, just to be thorough. You do this with people as you look to be affirmed in your identity, to feel safe with who you are. Being able to identify people 'like you' is part of a responsible survival strategy.

Here's another example of the RAS at work: You're thinking about buying a red car. You're excited about your choice. But all of a sudden, when you go for a drive, it seems as if there are *hundreds* of red cars on the road. Has everyone read your mind or have there always been red cars on the road that you just hadn't been *activated* to look for?

Your RAS ensures you find people who play the game in a similar way to your family and friends. Everyone understands which pieces of the game go where, whose turn it is and who are the likely winners and losers. Even if you're sick of playing the same old game because it's boring, or it might even hurt you or others, at least it's familiar and you know the rules. It's comfortable, or at least not uncomfortable enough to start asking questions about who set up the game to begin with and why you're stuck with this particular set of rules.

You choose to stay put in your beliefs and keep being 'yourself'. You might be comfortable enough to start recruiting others into your game. Your RAS recognises them as being familiar because they have a similar belief structure to you and they play by similar rules. You might bring a partner into the mix. This affirms even more that you are who you think you are because others think so too – and they choose you. This is powerfully enforced when you are in love and feel desired by another.

Finding people who don't sit well with your identity (and don't make you feel OK)

Sometimes, you venture into a completely different set of family rules. This can be a shock to the system and you're left asking, 'Who the heck are these people and where did they learn to play?' You start to think either *they* are nuts or *you* are going to go nuts playing this way. It's way outside of what your RAS is activated for. It's all just a little too different and who said you could change the game anyway?

Sometimes, you're desperate to get into a new game but because you don't know the new rules you return beaten and defeated back to the same old players and game board. Unfortunately your rules, like a bad smell, seem to follow you wherever you go. You can't see an opportunity to create change.

Does any of this sound familiar? Are you or others trying to change the rules of the game and it's creating stress, upset and confusion? This has certainly happened to me. I hope to have given you some hints about what could be generating some of your stress and upset.

Here's what happens next on your journey.

When your rules and identity aren't serving you. You feel stress. You ask 'Why?'

It's at this point in your life that you start asking the big question: 'Why is this happening to me?', 'Why do I keep ending up in the same old game with the same old players?'

We can assess our rules and decide if we want to live by them. If we find a way to rewrite them we can ask better questions. These better questions: When, Who, Where, What, and How are discussed in chapter 9.

Reader Activity

Do you have situations in your life, ways you react or ways others react to you and you simply can't understand why you keep getting stuck in this same place? Write them down – they will come in very handy once we get into the techniques.

You have been told who you are, how you fit in and the rules that apply to you by the people with the most influence in your life. Given this, could you be anyone else but who you are right now?

Summary

- There are rules to our game of life.

- We learn them before we are consciously aware we are doing so.

- We apply them, most of the time, without being consciously aware we are doing so.

- If we are lucky they work, if not we feel everyone else is cheating at the game.

- As we grow we have the potential to assess our rules and decide, 'Are these the rules I want to live by?'

NOTES

NOTES

Chapter 3

A simple example of 'The Set Up'

This chapter presents two examples of 'The Set Up'. They are a combination of clients' stories that I have simplified for illustrative purposes. As you read through them, consider how they might represent some of your own experiences. At the end of each example, note the type of questions asked by the characters. The questions are an important indication of whether the characters are ready to embrace change and move forward.

The game is set up

Mother: young woman from an abusive family background.

Father: her boyfriend who has a drinking problem.

They decide to stay together to raise their child (you) after an unexpected pregnancy.

You were born

Already there are so many ways this environment is fraught with potential stress and pressure. Yet those involved have made a decision to keep and raise you.

They teach you

You learn that Mum is often sad, Dad is angry and that's even before he starts drinking. You're taught that babies who cry get ignored or dealt with abruptly, especially when there's tension between Mum and Dad – which there is most of the time.

You create an identity

You try tears to get attention, that doesn't work. You try demanding, that doesn't work. You try throwing tantrums like Dad and that definitely doesn't work. You try being extra good and at least the shouting stops. You find that being quiet and good and mostly invisible are the best ways to get maximum positive feedback from Mum. That means Dad leaves you alone most of the time and isn't quite so mean. You don't feel safe but you know what to do to keep yourself safe. You are a 'quiet' and 'good' and 'invisible' person.

When we choose or operate from 'invisibility' or making sure that we slip under the radar as much as possible, it mimics the 'freeze' part of the stress response that works in part to make animals under threat 'invisible'. If they remain unnoticed the threat will pass.

You interact with others using this identity

When Mum takes you to see friends you hear people say you are a good kid because you never complain or get in the way, especially when the adults are drinking. In fact, you become very helpful, getting the alcohol from the fridge and then getting out of the way until you see a way you can be helpful again. You make sure no one gets upset. They don't acknowledge you unless they need something from you. Most people around you are quick to anger and rough in their language and responses. Being invisible and quiet works well.

You look for people who sit comfortably with your identity as that makes you OK

You find people that you can please because you already know you are really good at this and get good feedback. You notice you are especially good at doing this with people who drink or take other substances because you easily anticipate their needs and become very adept at resolving tension. You notice that many of your friends call you to come out because you are the one that gets them home after a big night out. Your friends also appreciate how well you help people calm down. You know how to do that well. You realise that your partner is most happy when you anticipate their needs. You decide it's really no big deal that they get angry and lash out because this is just part of the process – to you this is normal. You believe that if you are good enough it will all be fine. You are doing OK.

You settle down with someone that Dad really likes because they can have a drink together, and Mum can relate to because she knows about drinkers and so do you.

The person you think you might love drinks more. They had some issues that caused them to start drinking in the first place and if you can't beat them join them, right? The drinking becomes more and more difficult to manage but Mum put up with it so maybe you should too. Then there is a trauma in your partners' life. It makes your partner very, very angry and that's when the beatings start. And they don't stop. And they remind you of when Dad used to beat you after drinking and you hate yourself because you think you are not good enough. You have tried so, so hard but it is still your fault. Somehow you keep breaking the rules, you keep getting it wrong.

You think that maybe you deserve to be hit. It's not their fault, it's your fault – that's what they keep telling you and that's what you have always been told. For a long time you believe it's your fault – those are the rules of your game.

One day you can't stand it any more and get the courage up to leave. The trouble is all your friends drink so you feel uncomfortable around them as well. It's all the same feelings and stressors except now you are in someone else's home being unhappy. You may as well go back. At least in your home you have all of your own things around you. Anyway, maybe this time it will stop, your partner promised it would get better. It doesn't. You leave and come back a number of times. You ask yourself over and over, 'Why is this happening to me?'

Now, in comparison to the description above, see below.

The game is set up

Mother: young single woman from an abusive family background.

Father: her boyfriend who has a drinking problem.

On discovering she is pregnant she ends the relationship and goes to live with a loving and supportive relative who will continue to educate her while she raises the child.

You were born

Already there are so many ways this environment is fraught with potential stress and pressure, and yet this young woman has made some dramatic decisions to keep and raise you. Your Mum comes from a sense of hope and optimism with the support of a loving relative who has been a wonderful part of her life from the time she was small. She continues with her education and gets support in her new environment. You are her primary focus.

They teach you

You are taught that Mum sometimes struggles as she learns to handle her new situation but she is almost always loving and attentive to your needs. She has a mentor in her life that helps. You are taught that babies who cry get attention and are cared for.

You create an identity

You try crying and your hurts are soothed. You try throwing tantrums and that doesn't work as you are encouraged to deal with your anger and frustration by running around or doing something outside. You try being extra good and are encouraged when your efforts are rewarded with humor and cuddles and fun stuff. You find out being funny and helpful and creative gets maximum positive feedback from Mum. You know you can be cross and still feel safe because you know what the rules are when you are angry. You are a 'funny', 'helpful' and 'creative' person.

You interact with others using this identity

When Mum takes you to see friends you hear people say what a great kid you are because you find ways to amuse yourself so Mum can have some 'friend time'. You sometimes complain and get in the way but are encouraged to find ways to entertain yourself, to create solutions. Most people around you are fair and kind. You have got some interesting stuff going on in your own life. In fact, you become very good at thinking about what you love to do and letting other people know about it. You have friends who teach you about their families and who enjoy you being around. Lots of different people give you ideas about the world.

You look for people who sit comfortably with your identity as that makes you OK

You find people that ask you to 'think' and 'create' and you already know you are good at this. You get good feedback. You notice you are especially good at doing this with people who like to see the world from other peoples' perspectives. You have lots of conversations about the differences in people and what they bring to the world. You notice that many of your friends call you because they know they can trust you to get them home after a big night out. Your friends also appreciate how well you help them calm down and see things from a different perspective because you have learnt how to do that for yourself.

You settle down with someone that your friends and family really like because they can communicate without needing to drink. Mum can relax around your partner and you really appreciate that. You realise that your partner is very grateful that you can anticipate what they need. It is really no big deal that they occasionally get angry because this is just one of the emotions they express, not the only one. You also know that usually it has nothing whatsoever to do with you and they are entitled to their opinion. You are doing really well.

The person you love goes through a bad patch after a trauma in the family. They start to drink in an attempt to relax. They drink more and more and after a while you ask yourself, 'Does this really feel OK?' You discuss this with your partner and get an unusually negative response. After some thinking you ask yourself, 'WHAT can I do next? WHO can I talk to about this? WHERE can I go to get more information for what is happening in my relationship? WHEN shall I do something about this?' and 'HOW can I make a difference?'

As you can see from these stories, we are shaped, formed, influenced and trained to be who we are. Your mission, should you choose to accept it, is to see if you can break down your own story using the stages highlighted below.

Reader Activity

The game is set up

If possible, look at what was occurring in your parents' lives before you were born. Sometimes this may not be possible but write down what you know and also what you have been told and think you know to be true.

You were born

What do you know about the circumstances in your life after you were born? Do you know what was happening in your parents' lives at the time, their decisions around you and their relationship?

You create an identity

Regardless of what you know about these first two stages, you can look at the ways you were raised and the messages you were given about what type of person you should be or must be e.g. an obedient, silent child. Can you find ways that you have continued using the same criterion you did as a child to dictate your choices as an adult? For example, perhaps you don't answer back or are hesitant to voice your own opinions in case this gets you into trouble? There may be a lot of areas you can identify or just a few. Write them down as you will use them later.

You interact with others using this identity

I'm sure you have known or heard stories about the kid at school who got lots of attention for being the class clown or the funny kid. This identity works for them. Other kids like them and join them in their antics. Everyone feels comfortable and the child is affirmed with attention. We have all seen the child who gets attention with bad behavior. Keep in mind that although sometimes the attention we get is not positive, it achieves a desired outcome – to be seen and acknowledged.

Using these learned identities means we know where we 'fit'. How do you use your identity to stay within your existing circle of friends and family? Are you the peacemaker, the comic, the good child? A way to test yourself is to venture into a social circle that is very different from your own. Do you feel out of place or uncomfortable? Is it because your usual identity is not working in this new space?

You look for people who sit comfortably with your identity as that makes you OK

We tend to stay within our recognised comfort zones by finding others who share our values, beliefs and ways of being. This allows us to continue to be the same – even if we don't like it.

Reader Activity

Have you ever had an experience where you've met a person and known almost instantly, they are not someone you want to spend time with? Why was that? There may not have been anything specifically 'wrong' with them but you knew they'd never be part of your inner circle. If you can, identify what it is about others that makes them a 'fit' for you or not. This will tell you a lot about yourself and the lens through which you view your world.

Summary

- Rules of life are inherited from those who raise us.
- There are infinite variations in the rules.
- Whilst life may be unpredictable, the way we react to things is always according to our rules.
- Most of the time we don't know how to get new rules, even if we know we need them. We ask 'Why?'
- Sometimes, we find a way to rewrite our rulebook by asking better questions like, When, Who, Where, What, and How.

NOTES

NOTES

Chapter 4

There are no broken people (we're just playing with outdated rules)

At this point, do you have a sense that who you are is a direct result of who taught you to play your family game and what their rules were? Let's extend that out even further to say that the people who taught you are a direct result of who taught them and so on. When you think about how hard it can be to change things about yourself, your reactions, responses and interpretations, you can now get more insight into how difficult it might have been for the people who raised you to change their own feelings and reactions. This doesn't make excuses for anything, but it does offer you an opportunity to be more compassionate, especially to yourself.

We couldn't be a coherent, organised and productive society without rules. However the rules you're currently operating from do not have to be the totality of who and how you are. If the rules you live by are making you stressed and unhappy, or the people you love stressed and unhappy, you have the choice to review and discard the unwanted, unhelpful and outdated. Yes – you've followed the rules you were taught up till now, but if life is not going the way that you'd hoped and planned, you might be asking the 'Why me?' question all too frequently. You might now decide that the rules handed down through your family game no longer serve you.

As you contemplate this information, do you feel (as I did) a new sense of curiosity, even optimism about the future? Although you know some or all of the story of your past, the future might actually be yours to determine as you sift through and gather or discard. As you find new resources and techniques to create change within yourself, (like those in this book) your outcomes also change. You can change, everything can change, if that's what you desire.

One of the most profound things I learnt from Robert G. Smith[3], when I discovered his method of FasterEFT, is that there are no broken people. As he explains, '**There are no broken people, you are perfectly producing what you hold within you**'. You are simply operating from outdated rules that are no longer serving you.

What does this tell you about yourself? If you're not broken and you're simply producing what you know and doing it *really* well aren't you actually a success, already, just as you are? You might struggle with this idea because we spend so much time thinking we're failures.

The wonderful realisation this concept gave me was that if I *changed* the rules or feelings about the things I held inside of myself that I thought were true, if I uncovered my unconscious belief systems and dismantled them, I would be capable of something else. If we are not broken and are simply *perfectly* producing what we hold within us, then all we have to do is change what we hold within us and we will *perfectly* produce that.

I found this concept deeply moving. I no longer had to blame myself because I am not broken. Neither are you.

Given this idea, can you see that there is a solution to your stress and anxiety? If stress is simply a conflict between our expectations and our reality we must learn to understand what the expectations or rules are within us and decide if they align with the reality of our life. From there we can decide if this is actually enough for us to be happy.

Changing your internal environment to produce something else feels a whole lot more empowering than being a victim to beliefs you were unaware you even held.

Here's a simple example to illustrate how differing rules, beliefs and expectations create stress:

Your Boss looks at your work and gives you zero feedback. This makes you worried and stressed, as you believe 'no feedback' means your work isn't good enough. This has been going on for some time and your dream job feels more like a nightmare.

Now, examine your reaction: you expect feedback from your Boss but you're not getting it. This makes you stressed.

Your Boss, on the other hand, only comments on work that needs to be corrected or doesn't achieve its objectives. 'No feedback' is the Boss's form of praise!

After you look at this with fresh eyes, you could chat to your Boss about the lack of feedback and what that means to you. S/he might be surprised by how you perceive the situation since s/he has always done it this way and believes it's the way it should be done. You discover s/he is operating from a different set of 'feedback rules'. Is s/he wrong? No. Are you wrong? No. There are just different beliefs operating around feedback and when it should be given.

Being unable to change your Boss means you need to proactively find ways to adapt to your environment so that your expectations match your reality. When you change the meaning that 'no feedback' means 'my work is good' then you don't feel worried – then your reality falls into alignment with your expectations.

Just having this knowledge about different rules will help you manage your stress around the issue. You can decide to change the meaning you give the lack of feedback. It is within your power to do so. You are a 'meaning making machine'. **Choose your meaning, choose your rules, play your own game.**

How freeing would it be to play according to rules of your choosing rather than those handed down to you? YOU CAN. By learning and applying the ADAPTability method (chapter 16) the better you'll be able to manage your 'meaning making' and identify and disregard outdated beliefs. By the time you finish this book, you'll be able to change the meaning of any situation, write your own set of rules and let go of the rest. This way lies peace.

Reader Activity

- If you could completely rewrite your rules what would they be?

- How would your new rules transform your life now?

Summary

- You're not broken, you're just operating from a set of rules that no longer serve you.

- You can manage stress by addressing the meaning you apply to the stressor (trigger) and changing it if required.

- You cannot change anyone else; they have to do that for themselves.

- When you change what's within you the whole world and everyone in it looks different.

- The more you identify your 'meaning making', the easier it gets to change it.

NOTES

NOTES

Chapter 5

Meaning makes the difference

Let's explore the idea that our stress response is triggered by the meaning we give to an event, rather than the event itself. How can we use this proactively to manage our stress? How can we use 'meaning making' to positively impact our health?

'Reframing' to change meaning

This strategy which, in the fields of CBT and NLP is called 'reframing', is based on the principle that events or situations do not have inherent meaning – rather, the meaning is based on interpretation, which as we know, is made according to our particular beliefs, expectations and rules.

Some describe the reframing method as literally putting a different frame around the same picture to make the picture look different. Your rules and beliefs may have led you to use an antique frame – but a modern frame might make the picture much more appealing.

Take air travel as an example to get you thinking about the idea of perception, meaning and stress response: to some it's a frightfully stressful experience; to others it's an adventure in itself; for the crew it's all in a day's work.

The event is the same but the perception and meaning – and therefore the response – is different. Our perspective of stress comes directly from the meaning we apply to any given situation.

Cancer – a word laden with negative meaning for most people. But what about those who hear 'Cancer' and think of the star sign? With this interpretation, the disease doesn't even come into it.

Can you see the how the difference in our emotional response depends on the rules we apply to it, the frame we put round it or the meaning we give it?

You may feel that the meaning you give something and the stress it causes are difficult to separate, particularly if it's happening on an unconscious level. However, with practice you <u>can</u> change meaning and thereby reduce your experience of stress in a particular area.

Ignoring, denying, habituating

Changing meaning does not mean ignoring or denying the stressor. There's a big difference between ignoring stress and a stressor simply having no meaning or a positive meaning.

For example, a high level businesswoman who worked long hours under extreme pressure for many years eventually ended up in hospital with paralysis down one side. She believed she had suffered a heart attack or a stroke. She was actually experiencing a severe panic attack after ignoring years of signs and symptoms from her body that she was not coping. Despite the fact that her specialist made all the symptoms go away with a shot of a powerful sedative she continued to deny she had any other issue other than a physical one.

Like the businesswoman, sometimes we put our head in the sand and ignore the ways our body is letting us know we are starting to unravel. We do this out of fear of what we might find. If fear is a motivator for you to learn more about your stress, then use what you learn to change your belief systems. Give yourself a really big pat on the back right now because by reading this book and continuing your journey to discover more, you are in a great space to learn new skills and apply them. All of the people who really care about you and who want you to be around for as long as possible are so grateful for you making this effort as well!

How connected we are (or are not) to our body also influences our recognition of stress and our interpretation of the presence of stress or not. We physically process stress in different ways and our tolerance to stress fluctuates. Because we are amazing creatures and adaptation supports survival, we are also capable of habituating to stress. This means we are capable of determining if something continues to warrant being interpreted as stressful or not. Chronic stress may become our 'normal' and may continue unnoticed until our body starts to let us know there is a problem.

It is not only negative stress that we can habituate to. For example, giving a presentation at work might initially create many of the physical representations of stress such as elevated heart rate, shallow breathing and sweating. However, over time, with an increase in familiarity and some positive feedback, the situation could become pleasurable, we might even start to enjoy the spotlight and interpret all of those same feelings in a positive light. Now, it's become a positive stress.

Can positive stressors become negative? Yes, if we need to continually elevate the degree of any experience to produce the same feeling of positivity. Jumping off a cliff could give you a real adrenalin high. When you need to take greater and greater risks to get the same high such as using less equipment or knowingly going beyond your capabilities, it can become a problem. However meaning is every-thing, as you will see in the next section.

How thinking stress is bad for you – is bad for you

In recent years, scientists have begun to seriously explore the mind-body connection. Some fascinating research has been done in this area at The University of Wisconsin and Harvard University. Studies show that we are able to negate the negative impacts of stress by changing the way we think and give meaning to stress.

In their 2012 study, *'Does the perception that stress affects health matter?'*[4], Wisconsin Scientists examined the interaction between the amount of stress and the perception that stress affects health. Results showed that people who told researchers they felt stressed and believed it was negatively affecting their health were more likely to die prematurely in subsequent years.

The concept that what we believe about our stress has a direct impact on our health outcomes was reaffirmed in another 2012 study, this time conducted by Harvard's department of Psychology. *'Improving Acute Stress Responses: The Power of Reappraisal'* [5], found that positive feelings help protect cardiovascular health. 'We found that factors such as optimism, life satisfaction, and happiness are associated with reduced risk of CVD [cardiovascular disease] regardless of [other] factors,' said lead author Julia Boehm, 'For example, the most optimistic individuals had an approximately **50%** reduced risk of experiencing an initial cardiovascular event compared to their less optimistic peers.'

For more interesting insight, see health psychologist Kelly McGonigal's TEDGlobal talk, *'How to Make Stress Your Friend*[6]. In her presentation, McGonigal confesses that turning stress into a public health enemy through conventional talk therapies actually does more harm than good. 'The harmful effects of stress on health are not inevitable, ' McGonigal says, 'How you think and how you act can transform your experience of stress.' This is a great summary of what we are aiming to achieve by implementing the tools and techniques described in this book. By observing our thinking (consciousness) and acting to change it, our experiences of stress change, with positive benefits both physically and emotionally.

The link between emotional health and physical health

Unquestionably, our emotions have an impact on our body, more so if we think of stress negatively.

If we continue down the path of unchecked emotions and feelings and increased and prolonged experiences of negatively perceived stress, we risk harming our Nervous, Endocrine, Respiratory, Cardiovascular, Reproductive, Immune, Digestive, and Musculoskeletal systems. We succumb to health problems such as high blood pressure, cardiovascular disease, asthma, obesity, diabetes, headaches, depression and anxiety, gastrointestinal problems, Alzheimer's disease, accelerated aging and immune response suppression.

In 1998, the Journal of Occupational and Environmental Medicine[7], stated that individuals at high risk for stress have 46.3% increased costs to their health. (Depression tops that with a 70.2% increase to a person's healthcare costs.) In 2013, The Australian Financial Review's article 'Stress: The new workplace epidemic'[8] reported that Comcare, (the Australian agency responsible for workplace safety, rehabilitation and compensation), puts the average mental stress claim at $250,000 per person.

In the 1990s, a dramatic example of the holistic link between emotional health and physical health arrived, this time from a huge epidemiological study of 17,421 adults. The ACE (Adverse Childhood Experiences) Study[9], found an association between traumatic childhood experiences and disease. Many diseases, including the top 10 killers[10], correlated with unhealed emotional wounds. The higher the number of adverse childhood experiences, the higher the likelihood of diseases, disability and 'early death'. The ACE Study demonstrates unequivocally that early stress is a strong factor for developing health problems and that sustained stress in childhood results in profound lifelong impacts on the brain and body.

Over the past 25 years, research has shown time and again that our emotions are an important factor in immune system health. In a 1995 study, The HeartMath Institute[11] measured IgA (secretory immuno-globin A) levels in test subjects asked to feel care and compassion for five minutes. Then, several days later, subjects were asked to feel five minutes of self-induced anger. Researchers observed that positive feeling states boosted the immune system, while immune function could be suppressed for up to 6 hours after feeling angry for just 5 minutes. This is a startling example of the impact of emotions on physical wellbeing.

A forerunner in the field of mind body medicine and the science of psychoneuroimmunology, Dr Candace Pert Ph.D., a neuroscientist and pharmacologist, studied the interaction between mental processes and health. In her groundbreaking book, '*Molecules of Emotion*' [12] Dr Pert describes how our cells register the chemicals, hormones and neurotransmitters created in our body when we experience an emotion and that thousands of receptors in each cell receive information about our emotional state. Sadly Dr Pert passed away in September 2013 but research in this area continues to gather momentum worldwide.

The body is the unconscious mind

What does all this research mean in a practical sense when we are dealing with stress? Because our emotions are 'registered' by our mind and body, by isolating treatment to only the mind or only the body we can often observe a decrease in efficacy of treatment. My experience supports the idea that techniques that address aspects of the mind and body at the same time produce better results faster.

In some instances, my clients have been dealing with issues of stress and anxiety for decades. Many of them have sought psychological support. Many of them have used physical activity to deal with their symptoms. Both of these interventions are good but in many instances were simply not enough in isolation. It was not until my clients used the ADAPTability process and dealt with both the mind and the body concurrently that they achieved results.

The techniques in the coming chapters treat the mind and body as one connected system and generate solutions through a holistic approach. What happens in the mind also occurs in the body and visa versa. The opportunity this knowledge provides us is enormous and I believe predicts a transformation in the way we package and deliver healthcare in the future. We can see examples of this occurring already with the growth of multi disciplinary clinics offering not only the best in western mainstream modalities such as Chiropractic, but also the combinations of other disciplines such as Energy Psychology, Naturopathy, Massage and Exercise prescription. Once the exception, these types of holistic healthcare hubs are steadily becoming the norm.

In his best-selling book, 'Genie in your Genes'[13], Dawson Church quotes research into gene expression that illustrates that 'thoughts' along with 'meaning' directly influence the 'expression' of our genes. The research is a treasure trove of leading edge information that time and time again supports the synergistic influence between mind and body. This type of research highlights the importance of having some way to interrupt or support our mind and body synergy. In the instance of negative stress, our goal is to remove or at least reduce the ways we have 'learnt' the rules about stress and the habitual ways we deal with it. In this way we become the director of our emotional life rather than live at the whim of it.

Knowing how to deconstruct stress on both an emotional and physical level gives us the enormous potential of reconstructing the emotions, thoughts and feelings so that they support us physically and emotionally. We can positively influence our health using the <u>same</u> brain functions that are active when our health is being negatively impacted.

My goal for you is that you can actually transform stress and make it either work for you or have no negative impact.

Go to the tools and techniques chapters (13 – 16) to rapidly increase your ability to 'reinterpret' stress faster and more sustainably. Systematically using the tools and techniques will ensure it will take hours, not years.

Reader Activity

If you have something that represents a repeated conflict in your life involving another person, how could you reframe it to make it look and feel different to you?

Could you use this same strategy to reframe other things?

Summary

- Stress impacts every system within the body – especially if we believe it will.
- More and more research is discovering that what we think directly impacts our body, down to the gene level.
- What happens in the mind also happens in the body.
- You can use the body to address the mind and the mind to address the body.
- If you don't address both the mind and the body simultaneously results are muted.

NOTES

NOTES

Chapter 6

You – a hamster on the wheel of repeating rules

According to Albert Einstein, the definition of insanity is doing the same thing over and over again and expecting different results. Have you ever thought about how often you find yourself playing out the same old failed behaviours time and again and yet still you revert back to them? This happens to us all, no matter the promises we make to ourselves and to others.

We see the 'same old drama' dilemmas unfold in our lives – in our personal and professional relationships, our health, our financial goals, our 'to do' list, and our commitments to self. In fact, in every area where we experience challenge, our old patterns will show up. You may have promised yourself, 'This time, I will not allow my colleague to leave me with the bulk of work and take the glory', 'This time, I will not fall off the wagon after a week,' or, 'This time, I will be patient and keep my voice down no matter what the kids do.' There are lots of reasons that we experience the same stress and respond with the same behaviour over and over again.

Chemically, this is because by continually practicing our stress response, we strengthen it i.e. we get to a higher level of stress faster. The more we practice or 'think' our thoughts, the stronger they become. The stronger our thoughts become the more 'available' they are to jump into our thinking space and the faster our body jumps into a stress response as well. Anyone who has ever consciously observed their own escalation of stress will have noticed that as the stress feelings increase, the thoughts or ideas associated with the stress become more persistent. Eventually, these thoughts appear for no apparent reason but can immediately impact in a negative way. If we think of our mind as a super highway and picture our thoughts as vehicles, the thoughts we use frequently get the full six lanes of the highway because they require more space. Everything else gets the smaller lanes, paths, back alleys and goat tracks! This will continue until we learn how to redirect or garage the thoughts we no longer need or desire.

Emotionally we repeat stress behaviours because of the following types of set up.

Reader Activity

Consider how these situations might offer insight into your repeated patterns:

I want what they're having

We see a stress drama. We see what responses it provokes in others. We like those responses so we model (imitate) the stress drama. For example, our younger sibling cries for a treat and gets it. We learn that you can get what you want if you get upset. When we are older and interacting with others we continue to use this behavior to get what we want.

I never want to act like them.

We may design our lives around NOT being like someone we saw model certain types of stressful behaviour. However without tools to change our rules we do act like them anyway.

I'm out of control.

You hate yourself for doing it but it gets you what you want, so you keep at it.

I don't know what else to do.

We know we are playing by the wrong rules, as others have told us so. Yet we don't have the skills or information to change ourselves.

I have no choice.

It is impossible to change our behaviour because we believe it is 'so'.

I've always done it this way.

The incentives to change aren't there.

I give up.

We try to change, but we're not aligned with or supported by others, so we give up.

Summary

- We repeat behaviours even when we want to stop because we haven't changed our internal environment, rules and expectations.

- Even the best will in the world won't be strong enough to maintain a decision to change if the change we hope for is too different to what we have going on inside of us in the rules department.

- There are lots of reasons we do what we do but they always come down to what we hold within us. Most of the time we hold onto the rules we know because they are to do with 'belonging' and 'placement'.

- We can feel helpless to change.

- Change is possible.

NOTES

NOTES

Chapter 7

Having unrealistic expectations

We have discussed how we bring our rules, experiences, expectations and modeling to each situation and how this determines our responses over and over again. Learning to break the cycle is what this book is all about.

When emotions run high, many of us struggle to handle them. We often avoid 'taking ourselves on' at an emotional level for a number of reasons. One reason is 'denial'. Another is having unreal expectations – believing that we should be able to handle things and that something is wrong with us if we can't.

Our expectations of self and our ability to cope are often over inflated by necessity:

- Perhaps we have others relying on us and cannot let them down.

- Perhaps we have a huge goal and cannot let up for any reason.

- Perhaps we are in a situation we could never have anticipated and there is no turning back.

There's a lot of misinformation about how we are supposed to be and feel in our daily lives. Messages about what we should earn, how our relationships should be and what happiness should look like are everywhere. Through the media we're shown these ideals that alter our perceptions of ourselves and those around us. These first world problems become ridiculously difficult to manage, if this is all you have known.

I grew up believing in the fairy story of life. Positive and loving relationships were not being modeled to me, so Disney became my fantasy escape. My parents loved us but they were in a world of personal pain and didn't have the skills to focus on our emotional wellbeing. They did the best they could and it was a pretty good job. My siblings and I are healthy, contribute to society and love our own children. However, I chose the fairy story because it was in stark contrast to the relationships that I was exposed to. It gave me an escape and I believed that one day I too could find a prince who'd solve all my problems.

Growing up with a prince in mind has been one of the most detrimental things to my personal journey through stress and other emotions. It's been all too easy to attribute negative feelings and situations to the responsibility of someone else. I can *still* struggle when my partner of twenty odd years forgets I need a hug! These expectations set up internal struggles and judgments about who we are, how we're supposed to act and feel and what others are supposed to provide us with.

In many of the conversations I've shared with clients, we've all arrived at the same conclusion: When a new life chapter comes along, very little prepares you for the judgmental internal voice whispering, 'I should be able to handle this but I can't. What's wrong with me?'

I experienced this most strongly when I became a mother. Many new mothers feel this way – overwhelmed and like they are 'just supposed to know'. Often partners, as unskilled and unprepared as we are, presume that we should know it all as well. This doubt, guilt, worry and self-judgment comes at a time when we are most vulnerable. Many new parents seeking ways to cope with the stressors of parenthood have come to me to learn the skills to deal with themselves. I know these individuals are wonderful parents and that they'll use their newly learnt skills for themselves and their families, as I do.

Using my own experience to illustrate these points will help you to identify why it might be that you struggle to manage your emotions during times of stress.

Emotions vs. Feelings?

Emotions stem from the brain's release of hormones and neurotransmitters. When these reach the body, they're 'interpreted' based on our prior experiences and beliefs. Emotions are often considered 'beyond our control' and are chemically related to mental state and the way our individual brains are wired. Examples are affection, jealousy, fear and hurt.

Feelings, on the other hand, are physical sensations experienced in conscious awareness. They include, but are not limited to, things we can experience via touch, smell, sound or sight. Examples include shock, distaste, and a sensation of heat.

Because of the tactile nature of feelings they can trigger emotions. For example, experiencing a smell or hearing a piece of music can bring back a memory and the emotion of that time. Our feelings can be manipulated to create change within our emotions and visa versa. In the coming chapters you will learn not only to deal with unwanted feelings and emotions, but to actually use them as a resource to create change.

In my experience of being a new parent, feelings and emotions were all over the place creating lots of confusion and drama.

Experiencing overwhelm

I felt incredible love for my child, which was much more than I could comprehend. He was thriving, my partner was hands-on and things were 'looking good'. However, I was chemically mixed up, (I'd had a five-day labour and several interventions); my hormones were out of control and I was in a lot of discomfort (with enough stitches to sew a quilt). My overwhelming emotions were hard to identify – so new were they and so immense.

The love I felt for my child was the lifeline and in this way I was very, very lucky. Some parents don't feel this way when they meet their child for the first time. I surrendered my overwhelmed and confused self to be the best I could be for this incredible tiny being. I kept thinking, 'One day this baby will be a grown man and I could really easily stuff him up!' The burden felt huge.

I interpreted my emotions of fear, doubt and confusion as inadequacy. I interpreted my stress and anxiety as signs of weakness that would shame and embarrass me. When it came to big emotions, 'ignore and soldier on' was my type of modeling. Instead of recognising that in this new and extreme circumstance it was normal to feel this way, my modeling and interpretations of 'strength vs. weakness', based on my beliefs and experiences, silenced me.

I was also very conscious of wanting to reassure my partner that we were going to be OK. I believed I should be taking care of him as well. I told you I believed in fairy stories.

I put these indecipherable and contradictory emotions on hold as a coping mechanism. In hindsight I know that I numbed my emotions to avoid and deny them. Numbness is the feeling I chose to help me cope with what was happening in my life. I had a history of numbness so it felt familiar. Without new skills and knowledge we revert back to what we know.

(For those of you who think to yourselves, 'I don't feel anything', the numbness or emptiness you experience *is* an emotion you can work with. If your stress comes from a lack of emotion you can change it by manipulating your *felt* sense of your world.)

I didn't trust myself (or others) enough to discuss what was happening. I was confused because in my fairytale version this experience was so different. I felt a deep rage at not being given the *truth* about parenting and birth. I now know there is no single truth about anything except that which we believe at the time. Sometimes these beliefs are helpful and sometimes harmful. At that time, my beliefs and anger made me skeptical of the good advice that was coming my way. I isolated myself from support and became even more numbed out.

I continued to ask the wrong questions, 'Why is this happening to me? Why am I not happy? Why do I feel like a failure? Why didn't anyone tell me how hard it was going to be?' Lots of dead end questions leading to dead end answers and generating more faulty outcomes like blame, resentment, sadness and regret. Yet I loved my child, I loved my husband and we had the family I had planned. It was all a bit crazy, and by then I think I was too.

For a long time I thought it was OK to ignore things and that they would eventually pass. My determination to cope saw me escalate my numbness and denial. The trouble is that ignoring something often means it continues to accumulate – our body 'ups the anti'. Most of my clients speak of a gradual decline in their health correlating with an increase in stress. Our body will support us but only for so long. Eventually our nervous, immune and other systems start to struggle.

This knowledge is why getting out of the house more, spending more time with positive friends, allowing ourselves to be supported, watching funny movies, listening to music, playing sport or getting out into the sunshine, (basically doing the things we know we love and doing them often,) is so important. Through these 'felt' activities we are able to influence our emotions in a positive way. We also accumulate more positive experiences to draw on when the going gets tough.

Sometimes it does help to simply surrender to an experience. However there is a big difference between surrendering so you can learn from it and let it go verses surrendering *to* it – becoming a victim to it. (The Two Models of the World (chapter 10) looks at this idea in detail.)

Learning the lesson

I teach my clients that there is always an opportunity to learn from any experience. The experience is the lesson. Emotions are a lesson. Stress is a lesson. (Some of us need the lesson a number of times till we get the learning!) Our goal is to learn whilst we are in that feeling space. There is nothing more powerful than choosing to take a look at yourself when you are in the thick of it to get to the learning faster. When we spend time in that space we get to decide how we want to feel. Unfortunately, the space I was in had me believing it was decided *for* me, not *by* me.

I tried to address myself a couple of times – I failed so I gave up. I didn't have the internal resources at the time. I was a smart, talented, educated woman with access to information and I just couldn't do it. I now know that I was deeply entrenched in being a victim to my circumstances and getting a lot of 'poor me' scores on the board. Being a martyr is a very seductive and powerful persona.

You must persist with yourself. Keep looking for tools that work for you. Sometimes throwing everything at something is a great way to get results but this only works when you are in a strong state of mind. Sometimes trying to do everything at once just adds to your sense of inadequacy and overwhelm. I was a TCM practitioner, my husband a highly educated smart man, and between us we were clueless in the face of our emotions – talk about feeling inadequate! Sometimes, we are so far 'in' our stress we can't get perspective. We had too many tools and no idea where to start. It all felt so hard after our 565th night in a row of broken sleep.

As I continued down this line of no time, no sleep, no energy, no clue, it became harder and harder to imagine I might find a solution. Being in the victim state externalises your sense of control. When I was having the emotions of, 'it's bigger than me', I failed to realise that, 'it is me!' My feelings and emotions cannot be bigger than me when I am the one creating them.' I lost my sense of perspective to such an extent that I couldn't even work out were to start unraveling the mess that was me.

A couple of years later, as I learnt the tools I now teach to my clients, it became clear that this tendency to ignore the warning signs (given to me by feelings and emotions) is the part of us that tries to be 'superhuman' and lacks awareness of the mind-body connection. It also indicates how little we are consciously aware that we can manage our emotions by stimulating our feelings and visa versa.

I now know that you just start with the body and the strongest sensation, even if it's numbness.

Reader Activity

Do you have times that you know you are/were not coping? When are/were they? List them down to work on later.

Choose one of those times. Write down what your strongest emotions were and how you arrived at them.

Summary

- We bring our perceptions and beliefs to every situation, even when they're wrong.
- Numbness is also a feeling usually generated by overwhelm.
- Your feelings, or lack there of, are an opportunity.
- Asking the 'Why?' question keeps us in a victim state.
- Persist – this means you might fail. Persist anyway, just start with the strongest feeling.

NOTES

NOTES

Chapter 8

What happens in the brain when we're stressed?

I am not a neuroscientist and, I'm assuming, neither are you. Therefore, the description below is a simplistic one. For those readers who want to find out more about what happens in the brain when we're stressed, I've included further information in the resources section[14].

Simply put, there are three sections of the brain that are pertinent to our investigation into stress. The forebrain (front of the skull), the midbrain (middle of the skull) and the hindbrain (at the rear of the skull). Looking at the general role of these areas gives us real insight into stress and how to diffuse it.

The forebrain

This, the most sophisticated part of the brain, is where much of our logical processing happens. It is also the area of the brain that's highly activated when we are daydreaming, creating, socialising, relaxed and happy. It functions best when we're not stressed. In fact, when the stress response is in full swing, blood from this area is diverted to areas of the body involved in the flight or fight response such as the large muscle groups.

Some research indicates we can lose up to 10% of our capacity to make good decisions while stressed. Usage of this area of the brain is most apparent in animals with higher cognitive functioning, social and familial connections and those that can find creative solutions to problems. If we had to give this part of the brain an identity it would be that of a primate.

The midbrain

This is a different animal entirely. The midbrain is more like a cat. Have you ever noticed how cats are always aware of the exits in a room and are incredibly quick to find them when a threat is identified? This area of the brain is primed to be vigilant for danger and always aware of the surroundings. The midbrain continually assesses which response – either 'freeze', 'flight' or 'fight' – is the most appropriate and which is the best route out of a situation.

The hindbrain

The hindbrain is more like a lizard. It's purely about survival and responsible for our most basic and automatic functions. It includes the urge to fight, eat, breathe and breed but not much else. It reacts with the 'fight' element of the stress response and in extreme situations will promote extreme responses to get us out of danger.

Which part of your brain is in charge?

When the forebrain is activated and under positive creative pressure, we are capable of looking at the bigger picture, having greater perspective and empathy for others and working on our dreams and goals. Because this area of the brain works best when not stressed, we are better off to take a break and delay any decision-making if we know we are under strong negative pressure. The techniques in this book are designed to get you powerfully into your forebrain. You'll find the most creative solutions when it's highly activated.

When the midbrain is on alert and you're anxious, like a cat looking for the exit, you can calm yourself down with soothing physical contact, exercise or meditation. These physical measures stimulate the relaxation response allowing you to use more of your forebrain.

Interestingly, oxytocin aka the 'cuddle hormone' is also released during the stress response. This hormone directs us to seek out comfort from others. When they hurt themselves, children often freeze as they assess what's happened and the surprise registers, they then make a beeline 'flight response' to a significant person to share the experience and get support. Often, they are distressed and need cuddles and soft words of encouragement. These physical interventions directly influence the part of the brain that implements an escalation in anxiety and gives it soothing signals to calm down. Once calmed, children can often move on from the injury as the midbrain relaxes. Kids are not the only ones who need this. We are all children when it comes to the need for support.

If you think of your own stress responses, are you aware of a sense of escalation as the stress increases? This can often be noticed as increased physical agitation, irritation and frustration. We seek out support from others to help us move forward, conversing with friends, getting a massage, doing some physical activity. On some level, these activities mimic the 'hurt child'. As adults, getting appropriate support means we too can move on.

Supportive activities decrease the stress response and increase the relaxation response. As the midbrain is calmed, any escalation in the hindbrain decreases. Unfortunately these solutions aren't always possible: you can't always check out of a meeting to get a massage to calm your self down. That's why the techniques in the coming chapters are so valuable.

When the hindbrain is in charge, there is very little that can be done other than to get out of the way. A common example of the hindbrain in full flight is the tantruming two year old hurling themselves to the ground kicking and screaming. Parents who walk away or allow the worst to pass *before* they try to rationalise with their child are working with the natural functioning of the brain.

In some cases, when there's no real threat but alcohol or other drugs have altered our perception, our ability to rationalise our way out of senseless or violent acts is severely impacted and the brain slips into survival mode. Similarly, with enough negative experiences, our natural survival responses can kick in even when they are not warranted.

I had a client who experienced powerful feelings in her legs whenever we worked on strong emotional memories. She described it as a need to run away. There were many times in her childhood when running was a wise choice. Not running meant she got physically and emotionally hurt. As an adult, the triggering of any strong emotion provoked her survival instincts and she experienced these feelings in her legs. With ADAPTability tools, she used the intensity of the feelings as a gauge of her level of stress and implemented techniques to deal with it. *She used her body to understand her mind.*

This is a crucial distinction between the 'mind over matter' approach that has dominated our thinking for many years. We don't have to bludgeon our mind into submission with medication, electro shock treatment, aversion therapy or some of the extreme interventions we have experimented with over the years. The newer and more powerful tools use the mind and the body as insight into each other. Not 'force' but 'flow'.

Summary

- Your brain and body are connected chemically and through 'experience'.

- Your level of stress and your interpretation of that stress in any given moment can determine whether you are a creative genius or a violent offender.

- When we understand the way our brain operates we can create solutions using exactly the same 'hardware' and 'software' that interprets our experiences.

- Working with the natural flow of the mind is the best way to create fast change.

- You can use your body to influence and understand your mind.

NOTES

NOTES

Chapter 9

Resource States – Asking better questions to get better answers

When we talk about stress and it's influence, asking better questions is the key to discovering all the information we need to understand and change stress or any other negative emotion. Sometimes, despite the fact that the results we're getting in life are not what we want, going after a different result can take courage and commitment. Persist.

New results may not come without internal struggle as you navigate your way around 'meaning' and the rules you've always used as your guide to how the game is played. Asking better questions requires us to be willing to hear answers that may scare, hurt and challenge us. The prize at the end is being fully congruent and authentic, having questioned, checked and double checked the rules to your game and been satisfied with them.

As you ask better questions, you'll be sorting through your rules and realising many are outdated. Some of them you may have been aware of in the background and some only fleetingly, up till now.

These are the rules you inherited and have been running unconsciously. The great news is you get to choose if you want to keep them or not.

Ultimately, asking better questions allows you to redefine and re-experience who you can be in your world and how you can play your own game. Better questions allow you to quickly identify and understand where others are coming from in their question asking process. Understanding leads to growth and development. Asking better questions makes you the creator of your game not just a player in it.

Negative states, stuckness and asking the question 'Why?'

If you were really lucky you might have had an adult who knew all about better questions and taught you how to ask them. What a blessing. For the rest of us, the opposite may have been true. To a large extent we were simply taught and left with only one question. This question leaves us powerless and stuck in a *negative resource state*. It's the same state that ensures we struggle to change our perspective, to believe things could be different and to embrace change.

Because of the familiarity of this state internally and externally and the very nature of its effect on our ability to see the bigger game, we may very well believe this is as good as it gets – all there is for us in life and all there will ever be. We may look at others around us and at best feel a deep sense of inadequacy at our own inability to be like them or at worst ascribe negative reasons for them achieving differently, coping differently and feeling differently. We become incapable of perceiving there are options available for us as well.

Although unwelcome, this stuck state is familiar. It generally has a familiar result and follows a familiar course. It is therefore predictable and reliable. We often stay in this negative state because at least we can be certain of the outcome. Our deep desire for familiarity and predictability contributes to our stuckness. Our next thought, reaction and feeling is ruled by triggers from the past creating a domino effect. We can often accurately predict not only our own reactions but also those of others around us. We are caught in a loop of reactivity not creativity just as, so often, the people and situations in our life are too. The conversations with which we typically associate this kind of state might begin with, 'Every time I say…. they say', or 'Every time I do…. they do…'

Often, the results we achieve in a negative resource state are physically or emotionally painful. They can even be dangerous, like domestic violence or Saturday night bar fights or substance addictions. In their familiarity we find a sense of predictability that gives us a false sense of control even if the situation or ourselves are quite out of control. We persist in these situations for many reasons, financial and emotional. Often we stay in the negative state because we have just not reached the point were we are uncomfortable enough to make a change – a slow death by many small stressors that add up to disaster. It is this state that leads to frustration after frustration and stress after stress. The question associated with this state is the question that creates the conflict between our expectations of how things 'should' be and how things actually 'are' – the reality in our life.

The question associated with negative resource states is '**Why?**'

Many people (myself included) have spent large portions of life wandering around searching for the answers to their big questions using the 'Why?' question: 'Why did this happen?', 'Why did that happen?', 'Why him?', 'Why her?', 'Why them?', 'Why *Me*?' For many this has proven to be a stressful, frustrating and pointless waste of time, with hours adding up to weeks of life being held hostage to answers that may never be found. The answer might be, 'Why not you, when you keep asking the same questions, doing the same things and relating to yourself and others in the same way?!'

Why 'Why?' is the wrong question

Even if we know 'Why' it often doesn't change anything. Have you ever known 'Why' but it hasn't helped to change your feelings about a particular person, place or experience? Do you have a particular behaviour that makes you respond in a predictable way, you know exactly why it does this but you feel powerless to change your reaction? Phobias are good examples. If you have a phobia and you know that this started from a specific experience, does this knowing help to change the fact that you have to get as far away as possible from the source of your phobia?

When we ask the question 'Why?' and come from a negative resource state, all the answers exist outside of ourselves. This means all the *power* exists outside of ourselves. Some other person or situation holds the key to our state of mind, not us. Conversations associated with this might start with, 'I just can't help myself, it wasn't my fault she made me do it'.

When we ask the question 'Why?' we continue to feel helpless and powerless against the people, places and experiences that appear to be controlling our lives. In this state it's always, 'Her fault, his fault, their fault'. In this state we take little responsibility for our outcomes.

Negative resource states are very powerful states. They often exemplify a miserable, stressed and unfulfilled existence. Is this where you are coming from none, some or all of your time? Does the time you spend in this state correlate to the time you spend dissatisfied, unhappy and frustrated? Does the time you spend in this state inversely impact feelings of self-control, happiness and relaxation?

Asking better questions leads us to a positive resource state

So, what's our alternative? Well, if we want different results we need to ask better questions. When we ask better questions we return ourselves to a *positive resource state.*

In a positive resource state we have access to multiple tools both internally and externally, thereby exponentially improving our opportunities to change our responses to life. Therefore our results change as well. Whilst this alone can change the playing field of our stressed out anxious minds, with advances in our understanding of the way our minds work we can do *even more*. I explore this in more detail in the tools and techniques chapters.

Better questions are questions that either pull or push you towards a more positive outcome or at least an outcome that's different to the one you're used to. (Remember Einstein's definition of insanity?) This new result embraces and necessitates growth. It is a positive resource state. You could positively employ curiosity for example. This state may be quite different to the one you have traditionally used. The new state is better for you physically and emotionally, although it may be so unfamiliar that it doesn't feel great to begin with. The results you achieve from operating within this state contribute to self-empowerment, independence and growth. As Tony Robins says, 'If you are not growing you are dying'.

There are stages to our growth, which don't always appear externally obvious or prolific. Instead, we can be restructuring internally, incorporating or absorbing the 'new', a little like a gestation period. Often this state may appear as a stagnation period or even a period of death but it can be a time of recalibrating internally who we are within ourselves, to ourselves and to everyone else in our life.

This stage leads to viewing the world from a completely different perspective as we begin to view *ourselves* in a whole new way.

Reader Activity

Are there times in your life when the question 'Why?' has held you in limbo? Identify them.

Are there times when asking the better questions might have sped up your movement through a problem?

Summary

- Going after different results in your life can take courage.
- You may feel very uncomfortable along the way as you are challenged to adapt.
- Learning to ask better questions makes all the difference.
- Asking better questions makes you the creator of your game not just a player in it.
- Asking better questions enables adaptability.

NOTES

NOTES

Chapter 10

Two Models of the World

Using the 'Two Models of the World' provides us with a visual representation of how we might choose to live our lives. Imagine a blank page with a horizontal line through the middle. You have created a space 'above' and 'below' the line.

Below the line – the state of 'negative resources'

This is where the question 'Why?' is dominant. Using our game metaphor, this is the place where we cheat.

The question 'Why?' provides us with a never-ending source of possibilities to explain our discontent with life. When we ask questions such as, 'Why am I like this?', we look outside of ourselves to our environment, family and community seeking the answers and there's no shortage of evidence that provides us with the opportunity to blame.

Asking 'Why?' gives us ways to blame and avoid responsibility or change

We look to our family and see our father was an alcoholic and beat our mother; our parents were absent; we were the favourite until the new baby came along. We look to religion and find reasons such as original sin, invasion by alien virus or other indoctrinations. We look to the economy and blame the latest financial meltdown. We look to our addictions and blame the drug, the food, the pokies. We look back at school and blame the bullies or the teacher who shamed us in front of the class. We look to our finances and believe we can never be enough because our bank account tells us so. There are millions of ways we can answer the question of 'Why?' by looking outside of ourselves. However, if we remember the role of the RAS (which is to find what we are looking for) you will find what you are looking for and be able to continue to blame others, avoid responsibility and resist change.

In this space, negative emotions dominate. Our sole objective is to avoid our negative emotions. We look for substances (food, drugs) or activities (gambling, shopping, stealing) to avoid our emotions or at least distract us from them. Our 'felt' experience of the world moves us towards addictive or other behaviors to escape. When we have a 'distraction' experience, even if we only escape our emotions for a brief period of time, the pull towards it becomes stronger and stronger. We reframe it internally to have a positive meaning.

There are other ways we are manipulated by our feelings and emotions in this addicted space, which add to and compound its attraction. Consider a gambler: some experience or set of experiences led to the addiction. Whilst in the gambling environment, the lights, colors, sounds, people, atmosphere, loss of time, feel of the handle of the poker machine, smiles of the attendants, familiar faces, free drinks, food and the promise of a win all evoke a 'state' or 'trance' that makes the actual act of gambling even more attractive. These *feelings* help to distance the *emotions* that have driven the addict to their addiction and kept them locked in. These new feelings and emotions then become another part of this complex problem. The gambling persists, as does the avoidance of the initial emotions and feelings that provoked the need for distraction in the first place.

Our feelings and emotions are manipulated consistently and continually by our external world. Think of advertising, the glamorous interior of a casino or buzzing shopping centre. Think of the news, trashy and sensationalist magazines and TV. Think of horror movies!

So, what do we achieve by continuing to use the 'Why?' question to define ourselves, our experiences, our life? Living in the 'below the line' space enables us to stay exactly where we are – at the mercy of all the reasons, a victim to our emotions, experiences and memories. The perpetuation of the victim status disempowers and re-victimizes us again and again and let's us be right about our powerlessness. This might be the only time we actually feel powerful. If you have ever been driven by guilt into doing something for someone who played the victim card, you know how powerful the 'poor me' identity can be. Am I saying we should ignore the past and the ways we have been hurt? No. Am I saying it didn't happen and if you don't think about it it will go away? No. Am I saying it was all your fault? No. Am I saying that after reading this book you will have more control over your feelings and emotions than you have ever had before? Yes! Yes! Yes!

The externalisation of our control and power leaves little room for taking responsibility right here right now for what could happen next. We may not be able to take total responsibility for the events or circumstances that have lead us to this place, these relationships, these situations and the state of our life right now – however, what happens from *this* moment on is in our direct sphere of influence. The ways we participate, make decisions, choose to *feel*, and the ways we continue to respond from this moment on are absolutely in our power but only if we decide it is so, right here, right now.

There are benefits to continuing in this negative resource way of living and thinking. One of the most common benefits my clients report after choosing to explore this for themselves, is that living this way means it can never be *their* fault. Living within this belief system means we can blame someone or something else. We don't have to take responsibility for our feelings and reactions. We don't have to alter our environment. We don't ever have to face the challenge of ourselves being integral to the problem. This is a very emotionally manipulative and seductive space where we don't have to change and can continue on with our behaviors, beliefs, attitudes and projections.

If you can relate to living in the below the line space, rejoice! Recognising it is incredibly powerful! However, do you feel a little shocked or in grief by recognising these behaviours in yourself? Would it help if I told you I have spent a significant period of my life in the below the line space and still, every so often, drop down when I'm feeling really hard done by and sorry for myself? This is a very childlike state. It's the place kids go emotionally when they are miffed and need to blame their brother or sister. It's where adults go emotionally when the feel they don't have the resources, knowledge, experience or belief that it is no longer necessary. It occurs when adults are still children inside.

Above the line – the space for 'positive resources'

This is the space for positive emotions and the questions When? Who? Where? What? and How? Using our game metaphor, this is the place where we question the rules to make sure we're happy to continue playing by them.

This space illustrates the opposite of the below the line victim behaviours. In this space, we reach outside of ourselves to educate, grow, develop and improve ourselves. We manipulate our feelings to dispel emotions that do not serve us. When we go outside of ourselves to ask questions, it's with a whole different agenda. It's not to explain or excuse our behavior but to CHANGE it. We don't go outside looking to support what already exists in our life but rather, with a deep appreciation that we don't yet have all the answers and with an openness to be wrong about what we've always held true. We also feel capable of assessing whatever information comes in to see if it nourishes, supports and holds us in a loving and forgiving space.

Asking better questions gives us ways to grow and change

When?

With the question 'When can I do this?' we recognise that we have a choice to act:

- Q: 'When can I make some changes?' (A: 'How about right now?')

- Q: 'When can I have that honest conversation?' (A: 'How about right now?')

- Q: 'When can I take responsibility for my stress?' (A: 'How about right now?')

Who?

If we ask the question 'Who can I learn from?' we're looking for people who know something we don't. They might have knowledge that we'd like to incorporate into our way of behaving. For example, you might have a friend who's really good at relaxing to manage stress. They could teach you what they do to relax, and then the knowledge of how to relax *belongs* to you. It becomes internalised and a positive resource you can draw on to help you with stress.

Where?

If we ask the question 'Where can I find out more?' we're searching for more information and answers to our questions. We're also willing to accept that some of our existing foundations may be questionable. Answers to the question of 'Where?' might include a library, a support group, a friend you can trust, or an information site. When we ask, 'Where?' we do so with a curious mind.

What?

If we ask the question 'What can I do next?' we're acknowledging that there are possible pathways we can take in our lives and that every moment is an opportunity to make a decision. We are in the driver's seat and it's no longer the past that determines our behavior and reactions. It's no longer the future that forces our choices but a recognition of the moment we are actually in. The moment we are actually in is the only place we can make a choice for change. This doesn't mean we surrender our need to mitigate risk but it does mean we develop a faith in our ability for the worst to happen and for our response to be empowered, sustainable and good for us.

There are other powerful above the line questions. One of them is THE power question and it's coming right up in the next chapter.

Reader Activity

Here's where I make an exception to the 'Don't ask 'Why?' rule'. When you've decided you're determined to make changes and need to look at the beliefs, behaviors and habits that lead to your stress, you may ask 'Why?' In this situation you are choosing to explore and not to blame.

Ask yourself 'Why am I stressed?'

Write down everything that comes to mind, no matter how obscure, strange or obvious. If you're able to blame mum, work, the dog, your job, your finances etc. make note. Every scrap of it is great information to focus on when we apply the techniques in the following chapters. You will get the greatest and fastest change when you're able to focus. You can use this information to make your breakthrough and never make excuses again! Don't get yourself in a bunch over this if you have no idea why you are stressed – there are techniques for that too and this comes to light when we discuss the power question.

Summary

- We can live below or above the line, but it is our choice and our choice alone.

- We can directly influence our emotions using our feelings to move us above the line or to keep us below the line.

- There are benefits to living below the line – we get to be victims and it can never be our fault. We also get to continue our addictions. This way of living is self-perpetuating. We allow our feelings to perpetuate our way of being.

- The most powerful difference between 'above' and 'below' is the questions we ask.

- There are benefits to living above the line – we get to be solution finders and leaders. We also get to do a lot of the things we love because we know that doing so sustains us. This way of living is self-perpetuating. We use our feelings to manipulate our negative emotions.

NOTES

NOTES

Chapter 11

The Ultimate POWER Question –
'How do I know I have a problem?'

Asking the question, 'HOW do I know I have a problem?' leads us down an incredible pathway of exploration.

Initial answers to this question may point us to the external world for evidence, dipping us 'below the line'. If your answers are like those below, just go with it and write them down:

'I know I have a problem because my partner, co-workers and boss tell me so.'

'I know I have a problem because the Doctor told me my blood pressure is high.'

'I know I have a problem because there's no money in the bank account.'

'I know I have a problem because I cannot focus.'

These answers are good but they provide external references to our problem. They are only *symptoms* of the problem.

The only way we really know we have a problem is because we *feel* it and *believe* it to be so.

Let me give you some examples that illustrate the difference.

I had a young client who was self-harming by cutting herself. Everyone around her knew she had a problem including her teachers, parents, siblings, psychologist and friends. She didn't believe it was an issue. She continued to self-harm despite what everyone else thought and despite all the evidence presented to her, even despite the very real possibility of her being institutionalized. All these people wanted to 'take away' the only resource that *'felt'* like a solution to her.

Logically, you and I know there is something much deeper at play here. However, until that young women determined for herself that the 'pain' of self-harm was worse than the pain of 'dealing' with what was really going on, she refused to stop. She didn't believe there was a problem and so for her there wasn't. In fact, there was a lot to gain – cutting gave this client *relief* from her internal environment, her feelings and emotions. Everyone else saw 'problem', she *felt* solution. Additionally, this behaviour gained her a lot of attention. The attention was obviously both positive and negative, but it was all attention. The shock and revulsion, the fear and pity, all the appointments and questions achieved something for this client, which was to finally be given some acknowledgement that she was in trouble. The self-harm was a very effective means to an end so she was reluctant to give it up.

Another client I had bankrupted his family business through gambling. His partner reached out to me in desperation and he agreed to come to a session. When I asked him if he had a problem, his response was that he didn't *feel* it was a problem because he *believed* he could always go out and earn more money. His partner was dealing with the loss of the family home, two small children and the debt collectors all on her own, yet he resented her for trying to embarrass and manipulate him into changing his behaviour. Again, what this client was avoiding was more painful than what was actually occurring.

These are extreme examples but in my work I see these examples all the time. Any solutions for these clients had to do 'better' than the ones they had found for themselves: cutting and gambling.

Remember the highly paid businesswoman who ended up in hospital thinking she'd suffered a heart attack or stroke? She believed there was only a physical problem because she was incapable of dealing with herself on an emotional level. She had no skills in this area and unfortunately was in a toxic work environment that celebrated aggression, strength and a 'never say die' attitude. This environment offered her no opportunity to learn about resource states or better questions. Not until much later in her journey and after many years of struggle was she able to see what she'd been doing internally and take responsibility for it. She now runs educational programs for people in her profession, and guess what? Many of her colleagues were suffering in the same way.

Self-harm comes in all shapes and sizes

Addiction or any other type of negative behaviour that puts you or others you love at risk, any internal negative judgment such as ridiculing or disparaging self-talk, (like when you say to yourself 'I'm an idiot'), are all examples of self-harm. Unfortunately, until we recognise them as such they are not a problem. Until we ask ourselves do we *feel* this is a problem inside of ourselves because we experience it through an emotion, a physical sensation, a numbness or a pain (to mention a few), we cannot shift into finding resolution.

Unless it is a problem for <u>you</u> it's not a problem

When we actively ask, 'How do I know?' and go looking for tools and positive strategies for growth to enable us to deal with stress and other behaviours, things will not change. When we are dissatisfied, fed up or disappointed by how we are feeling, <u>then</u> there is an opportunity to change. Then and only then can we move towards real and sustainable solutions.

What this indicates is that we have *no chance* of helping others resolve their problems unless they are ready, willing and in agreement about their problem. You can only deal with yourself, your internal environment, your feelings and emotions – not anyone else's. You might think you know what someone else is feeling but you can only approximate this based on your experiences. We can empathise but we cannot *know*.

So don't deal with other people's stress, deal with your *own* feelings about your own stress. Don't deal with other people's addictions, deal with your *own* feelings about your own addictions. Move away from them, they may not have decided there is a problem yet (or ever). Move into yourself. Within you is where you have the most power. Within you is where you can check-in to see if you are using positive or negative resources; asking power questions or dead end questions; operating above or below the line.

When you're determined to heal you first, the Ultimate POWER Question, 'How do I know?", can change your life.

I appreciate this concept might be challenging. A common question I hear is, 'What about children dealing with stress who don't have the same control over their lives as adults do? Can they really be expected to ask better questions and resolve to change?' In the case of children, I suggest that we teach them how to ask better questions and offer ourselves as their positive resource model, giving them skills, opportunities and mentoring about different ways to experience their lives.

In the same way, we can be the adult for the child within us.

Heal yourself first and then what you bring to the world is a healer.

Summary

- The only way we really know we have a problem is because we feel it.

- We have no chance of helping others resolve their problems unless they're ready.

- Heal yourself first and then what you bring to the world is a healer.

- Deal with yourself first and then teach others by example.

- When you get stuck, ask yourself 'How do I know I have this problem?'.

NOTES

NOTES

Chapter 12

The faster we become aware the faster we can repair

Wouldn't it be great if we were quickly aware of the messages our body sent us to alert us to what it perceives as danger or stress? As we became aware of our mind and body we are in CHOICE.

We gain power by bringing awareness and focus to our feelings and emotions.

The potential to find what we 'set' our minds to look for is a powerful tool of control and discovery. Activating the RAS by giving it something specific to detect is a great way to develop clarity and focus and to reset what we believe about the world.

For example, if you're someone who believes fundamentally that people are not happy, you could set yourself a task to count the number of smiling people you saw in a day. If you set out anticipating smiles, you will find them in record numbers. You could do the same thing with small acts of kindness. Would doing something like this change your perception?

The following exercise is about finding your stress experience and noticing what it is for you by paying attention to your body. It will give you a way to speed up your ability to deal with the impact of your emotions (how you 'feel' them). The faster you're able to recognise your stress response, the faster you'll be able to take the measures required to change or alleviate it. Rather than being at the mercy of your feelings, you can use them as a resource to solve the problem. What you 'feel' and 'experience' in your body of your emotions then becomes a primary indication of how well you are dealing with them.

You – the non-judgmental observer of your emotions

Besides the benefit of increased awareness, there is another: an awareness of our emotions allows us to separate from them rather than 'being' them. If we can describe our emotions, it means we are able to observe them as separate to ourselves. We can certainly 'own' our feelings and emotions and describe them as ours – 'my stress'. However, your stress cannot own you. Your stress cannot make the same claim – 'my human'. Many of my clients express real relief when they become aware of this. We are not our emotions; our emotions are simply one *expression* of ourselves. When we use the expression, 'I am stressed', it implies, 'I am stress'. But the truth is, we 'feel' stress in our body through various physical sensations – a tightness in the chest, dry mouth, churning stomach etc. The stress is not 'us'.

Seeing your emotions as something you 'do' rather than something that 'does' you gives you greater capacity to change. Understanding that your feelings are just an expression of your emotions means you can change them as well. You are not broken just operating from some outdated rules.

Many of my clients are very angry with their body, especially those who experience chronic pain or health conditions. They have forgotten that the mind and body start out as our servants. Over time, often without our conscious awareness and direction, they start to take over and become our masters. At this point we believe we are at the mercy of our mind and body (this is a below the line type of thinking). There is often a sense of rage and despair at this situation. What's required are techniques to take back control.

With practice you can more and more easily become the *observer* of your feelings rather than a slave to them. Know that over time, as you build your 'awareness' muscles, you can choose to see your mind and body as a faithful partner who stepped in to take over the kingdom when *you* abdicated the throne for some reason.

Over time, as you practice observing your stress as separate to you, an expression of you, a symptom of yours, you can choose to be the non-judgmental observer. Notice the stress experience and then implement your tools to disconnect from what have become the mind and body's automatic responses. You will become an expert at this, connecting in within seconds, as you become more and more familiar with how you 'do' your stress. When you can observe your feelings you can change your emotions. When you change your emotions you change everything.

Over time and with the application of the tools, my goal is that you let go of the hook of needing to 'check out' thereby allowing your emotions to rule you rather than the other way around.

Disassociation – Are you checking out?

'Disassociation' is something many of us have used at times in our lives when we have simply become too triggered, too stressed, too overwhelmed to cope. Our mind perceives disassociation as a solution to the emotions we're experiencing, much like the gambling and self-harm mentioned previously. Our mind then determines that this solution works because we perceive that our stress response in the body decreases and stops sending the danger feedback signals.

The mind then implements the 'disassociate' solution whenever it perceives that degree of emotion again.

Sometimes, we disassociate whether the emotion is a good or bad emotion. Our mind makes no judgment around what constitutes good or bad. Instead, the mind simply distinguishes the degree of feeling that the emotion provokes. The mind then relates back to an experience of a similar degree of emotion that at that time we interpreted as unacceptable. It then goes to the winning strategy that had previously taken you away from the danger of feeling too much. Often, when we think of people disassociating, we think of an extreme situation. The reality is that what is extreme for you and I and someone else can be completely different things. For many of my clients, checking out has become so common they are completely unaware that it can happen within a normal context; like a conversation where they have not been able to answer a question and this provokes emotion.

I want you to check into how often you might be checking out. If you find it's often, then the more techniques you become familiar with and implement, the greater the result you will achieve. There might be a whole life out there waiting for you that you've not been present for. Sometimes it's helpful to ask someone who spends a lot of time with you and that you trust, whether they feel you check out and when, where and with whom you do it. Notice I didn't ask 'why' you might be doing it. It doesn't matter, you might know or you might not.

If you have trouble focusing on your *felt* experience of stress, remember that numbness and disassociation often go together. Notice how you know. Ask yourself, 'How do I know I am stressed… sad… angry… disappointed? Am I numb? How can I tell I am numb?'

Reader Activity

Read through these instructions first, then find 15 minutes or more to complete the exercise. Write down what you observe, notice and feel. If you don't continue to read after completing the exercise, keep your notes. Whilst you take a break from reading, try to keep practicing noticing 'how you know' you are stressed.

Think about your stress.

I want you to sit quietly and give yourself a chance to focus, to pay attention to you. There is no right or wrong in this exercise. If you are currently experiencing stress, this will be easy. If you are currently relaxed, choose either one thing you know triggers your stress or one way you know how you *feel* your stress and focus on that. Now feel it as though it was happening right now. Pay close attention.

Can you locate your stress somewhere in your body?

You might have an awareness of its location. Perhaps you feel something in your chest area. Perhaps it feels like it is right below your heart and more on the left than the right, or perhaps your stress is in your neck or shoulders, or perhaps it feels like it is just outside your rib cage or behind your eyes.

Notice what you 'feel' in terms of sensation.

Some of the ways my clients have observed their stress include feelings of tingling in the legs; pins and needles in the hands; a shroud over the face; a heavy load on the shoulders; a tightness in the chest; a tight band around the temples; increased temperature; perspiration; shorter breaths; a raised heart beat. As you focus, perhaps you can get an idea of its texture. Does your stress feel tight or sharp, thick or foggy?

Other ways you might notice your stress

Perhaps you become aware that your stress has a shape – it could be like a blob or a brick. Does your stress have its own color? Perhaps you notice a sound like a ringing in your ears or sense a particular smell? Don't judge, just notice whatever it is that you become aware of as you pay attention.

Noticing takes practice

This may be a little hard at first. It may feel like a *logical* exercise rather than a *felt* exercise. We live so much of our lives in our heads that we forget we are attached to a body. We forget our body carries our stress on our behalf.

Write down your notes.

Summary

- The faster we become aware the faster we can repair.
- We gain power by bringing awareness and focus to our feelings and emotions.
- Step back far enough and you can become the non-judgmental observer of your emotions.
- Noticing what is happening within us takes practice.
- Our body is our greatest ally.

NOTES

NOTES

Part 2

Tools and Techniques

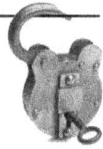

Chapter 13

Introduction to The Quick Tap

This chapter will help you to take the awareness you've developed around 'how you know', and use it in a very focused way to create change.

Used correctly, the technique can create change in minutes not hours. The more you practice, the better and faster you'll become and the greater your confidence will be. Using this technique correctly and systematically has impacted even the most severe experiences of trauma and illness.

Please note, a severe trauma or overwhelming emotion is not the place for you to start when you're on your 'L' plates with this technique. When you're a beginner and working by yourself it's best to choose experiences/emotions that you would rate no higher than a 5 or 6 on a scale from 0 – 10. (Your goal is to get them down to a rating of 1 or below.) When you begin with a less intense experience, you'll soon gain confidence to take on the bigger issues. Frustration with sitting in traffic is

an example of a minor stressor, whilst dealing with traumatic memories is an example of a major stressor that, as a beginner, you might want to seek assistance with.

Read through this chapter, and then put the technique into practice for yourself. The sooner you start the sooner you can manage and then create change in your life.

There's a big difference between *managing* our emotions and *changing* them. For now, management alone is a brilliant outcome. Management is also useful when we're in a situation where we can't get too emotional, for example when we're out in public or in a meeting.

Tapping changed my life. It can do the same for you. My hope is that you will *transform* the way you experience stress and reduce the negative impact it has on your life. I would love for you to transform it to the extent that it's no longer recognisable. This takes practice, but is possible within minutes once you get proficient. Whether you decide on management or complete change, congratulations on your choice to play a different game within yourself and out there in the world!

The Tapping exercise I'm about to show you is from Robert G Smith's Faster Emotionally Focused Transformations (FasterEFT) methodology. FasterEFT is my personal preference and style, however any style of Tapping is powerful. Kim Jewell also describes this technique, called 'The Quick Tap', in her e-book *'From Stress to Success'*[15].

In a quick metric from my practice, I have close to a 95% resolution rate for my clients with less complicated problems within one to three sessions. For more complex cases the rate is closer to 95% over six sessions. By resolution I mean that the problem that was strong enough to prompt the client to seek help, no longer exists in the same way. The circumstances and people that might have contributed to the problem may still be the same but my client's response to it has fundamentally transformed. This is a powerful technique. However, as I say to all my clients, 'the proof is in the pudding'. You have nothing to lose and a whole new you to gain.

What is Tapping?

Tapping is using your fingers to lightly tap on specific points on your body. In FasterEFT the points used are at the end points of your inner eyebrow above the nose, beside your eyes, under your eyes on the ball of your cheek, at the collarbone and you also squeeze the wrist. See page 129 for a diagram of the points. You circuit through these points until you have achieved your desired result. As a general guide you tap on each individual point for as long as you feel you should, (start with 7 – 10 taps per point) and then move to the next one until you get a feel for it. You end with the wrist squeeze.

See the diagram below or go to www.drlindawilson.com to see my Tapping video[16]. Notice that I use both hands to show the points on either side of the face. You can use both points on both sides, just one side or cross over sides, whatever is more comfortable for you.

Don't over think this, just try it and notice how your awareness of 'how you know' changes.

If you've come straight from the previous chapter and you've focused your mind to identify 'how you know' about your stress or problem, proceed to the next step. If you've had a break since reading the previous chapter, finish reading this section, then repeat the previous exercise so you're aware of 'how you know'. If you have awareness of multiple 'how you knows', for example a tightness in the chest *and* heaviness in the head *and* churning in the stomach, choose one of the feelings/sensations. Write the others down so you can move on to them later.

The Quick Tap

1. With your eyes closed, pay close attention to one specific 'how you know' only.

2. Associate to (feel) that one thing as strongly as you can. Make it as real as you possibly can, as though it is happening right now.

3. Notice 'how you know' and give it a score out of 10.

4. I want you to imagine a tree in front of you. For some reason we don't need to know or worry about, the tree falls over and all the roots come up out of the ground. What happens to a tree with no roots? That's right, it dies.

5. Open your eyes and keep them open while tapping.

6. Now start tapping between the eyebrows.

7. As you tap, pay attention to the sensation of the tapping on your skin, keep your eyes open.

8. As you tap, say out loud, 'Let it go'.

9. Move to the side of the eye and start tapping.

10. As you tap, pay attention to the sensation of the tapping on your skin, keep your eyes open.

11. As you tap, say out loud, 'Let it go'.

12. Move to under the eye, right on the ball of the cheek and start tapping.

13. As you tap, pay attention to the sensation of the tapping on your skin, keep your eyes open.

14. As you tap, say out loud, 'Let it go'.

15. Move to the collarbone area and start tapping.

16. As you tap, pay attention to the sensation of the tapping on your skin, keep your eyes open.

17. As you tap, say out loud, 'Let it go'.

18. Move to the wrist. Encircle the wrist with your other hand and squeeze gently 3 or 4 times.

19. As you squeeze, say out loud, 'Safe to let it go'.

20. Release your wrist.

21. Take a big deep breath.

22. Blow your breath all the way out and say, 'Peace'.

23. Close your eyes and go to a great memory. Choose a memory that fills you with joy, love or happiness. It could be anything, a great coffee; the last time you kissed someone with passion; a place that makes you feel safe or happy – whatever you want as long as it is good. Notice everything about it; the colors; the temperature; who else was there; the sounds etc. Make all your positive feelings stronger. Spend some time there. Notice 'how you know' how good it feels. Really feel those good feelings.

24. Take a big deep breath, say, 'Peace' and open your eyes.

25. Now, go back to the 'how you know' of your original problem. Stay with the feeling you chose to focus on. Pay attention.

26. Notice if it has changed in intensity in any way. It may have increased or decreased. It may have moved location. Just pay attention.

27. Score the feeling out of 10 and write down your new score.

28. Do the tapping exercise again.

29. Don't worry about the tree visualisation – this is only required at the start of your tapping sessions.

30. Your goal is to get your score down below a 2.

Once you have done this for the initial problem you chose to focus on, go back to your list of 'how you know'. Choose another. Tap through this one as well and so on until you are done. Be thorough, be persistent, be your own best friend and encourage yourself to stick with it.

You might notice a couple of things as you go through this exercise. For example, when you change your feelings or the 'how you know' of one problem, some of the other feelings you associated with it might change as well. You might have gotten a reduction in the tightness of the chest *and* the churning in the stomach for example.

This is because as we change one aspect, our mind loses the strength of connection between them all. When we change and weaken one link as part of a chain of experiences or feelings the 'mind' loosens its grip on the maintenance of the others.

When you get to the stage where you feel satisfied you have reduced the feelings or sensations to a 1 or below, check to see if there's a way you can bring your initial feeling back. Now don't freak out here – many of my clients express dismay when I ask them to do this exclaiming, 'I don't want to bring it back!' It's important to do this part of the process because we need to be thorough. The intention is to test that the 'how you know' or the feeling you have been working on is truly gone. . . If you can bring the feelings back, notice how you did that. Did you see something inside your head or hear something from that time? Notice 'how you know'. Tap on the feelings or sensations or thoughts that come up when you do this using the technique. When you're satisfied that you've reduced the feeling or sensation down to a 1 or below and cannot bring it back, pay attention to your whole body. Do you feel different? More relaxed? More grounded? More comfortable in your skin? Tired? Elated? Surprised? Pay attention and write down your score.

After a couple of rounds you should be able to see a shift in your scores.

This is a very simple explanation of a single exercise and practice within FasterEFT and a powerful tool for you to quickly make changes for yourself. On its own this single tool can transform your experience of stress as well as other emotions. However like the gym – the more you use it the better the results, so build those tapping muscles! And as with gym equipment, there are many more tools and techniques I use in my own practice in any given session.

Some people find it helpful to keep a Tapping journal.

To find out what is actually happening when we tap, keep reading.

Summary

- Watch the video first and follow along to gain confidence.

- Become familiar with the location of the points on your body.

- Follow the sequence carefully to begin with. You can experiment with variations later.

- Don't be tempted to tackle the really big stressors in your life to begin with. Get your confidence first or get trained help.

- If you feel you're not getting results, I encourage you to find a Tapping Practitioner through the resources section at the back of the book.

NOTES

NOTES

Chapter 14

Dissecting The Quick Tap technique

The technique is structured in a very particular way to get the best results. Go to www.drlindawilson.com and follow the link to see me discuss this information.[18]

Associating with the feeling
(Tip: the more real you make it feel, the faster it goes)

The aim is to get the mind and body focused on the target for tapping by imagining the strongest experience of our problem. To make it as real as we can, we feel what was felt; see what was seen; hear what was heard; smell what was smelled. Closing our eyes whilst getting associated with our problem helps us bring it into focus.

If you've experienced this problem many times, choose the time that evokes the most emotion and focus on that. It's the degree to which we are able make our problem feel real that makes the biggest difference to our results.

Visualising the dying tree

Once we have associated and scored our feeling out of 10, we use the falling and dying tree visualisation. The mind searches for connections between things as a way to organise our world. We can use this habit to our benefit and create change. By using the thoughts feelings and images you have associated to your problem and putting them together with the tree, it sends the mind a powerful message that those feelings will now suffer the same fate as the tree.

We give the mind a visual image – the tree – and an auditory command – 'it dies'. The tree dies because it becomes completely disconnected from what is keeping it alive. Since our mind has connected the tree and the problem, it's like shorthand for 'Problem equals tree. Tree dies. Therefore problem dies.'

Tapping

During tapping, we focus on the sensation on our skin while saying out loud, 'Let it go'. Opening our eyes helps as we interrupt access to our feelings. There are five things happening here:

First, we are triggering a relaxation response in the anxious mid brain via physical touch and using a soothing voice.

Second, we are issuing an audio command to 'Let it go'. As the mind goes searching for what to let go of, it's aware of the problem most recently associated with and all the 'felt' aspects of that problem. Through the suggested link, and the activation of the feelings associated with the problem, the mind utilises the command to 'let go' in relation to those feelings and that problem and let's go of those.

Third, we are interrupting our association to the problem by focusing on the tapping sensation, keeping our eyes open and using the phrase 'Let it go'. All of these contribute to disconnecting and destroying the connections we have to the problem – both real and perceived.

Fourth, the tapping has a physical influence on the meridian system. The system is triggered to energetically restore balance to the entire system.

Fifth, we squeeze the wrist and take a big deep breath. The breath tricks the brain into being relaxed (as we only take deep breaths when we are relaxed). The mind is being further and further convinced that there is no problem as all the felt sensations of the problem leave the body with the command to 'Let it go'. We blow the breath all the way out, again reinforcing the relaxed state.

Last, we say 'peace' out loud. This is another auditory instruction to pay attention to the new state, which is more peaceful. The mind will go looking for the peace we have mentioned because it is a meaning making machine. It will find peace because we have supported it to do so. The whole concept of peace and what it means to be peaceful is recognised by the forebrain so again, this instruction is easily obeyed, as we are now feeling peaceful.

Remember the super highway? Through this process we are reducing down the available lanes for the problem to travel on.

What looks so simple is actually layered with instructions, commands and intentional associations for the mind and body. This is the *new path of meaning* we want to give the mind in relation to your problem.

Summary

- Your problem – the tree – it dies – be calm (touch), be calm (voice)
- Let it go (command)
- It's safe (reassurance)
- Deep breath in (mind relax) – releasing breath out (mind relax)
- 'Peace' (naming the new state).

NOTES

NOTES

Chapter 15

How Tapping works

When we tap, after focusing our mind on specific negative emotions or physical discomforts and issuing verbal and visual commands, we guide our mind-body system to let go of physical/emotional connections and outdated associations and beliefs.

Though we do not yet know exactly how it works, we do know that it works on a number of different levels, which is why it's so effective.

Soothing the anxious midbrain

When we manage our emotions with Tapping, we're working to reverse any escalation in the stress response. Furthermore, we're aiming to increase the relaxation response.

The resources (including blood/oxygen) that have been shunted into the large muscle groups to prepare to fight or flight, are again freely available and the hormones and chemicals associated with stress (such as adrenaline) are processed out of the system. The midbrain is soothed and calmed by a gentle voice and physical touch (remember the hurt child who froze then ran to be soothed?). By calming the midbrain down we move back into being able to use the forebrain. From this space we can more easily manage and act to deal with our feelings, emotions and the conditions in our environment that might be creating our stress.

Creating measurable and sustainable change in the brain

Scientific research shows that changes in the brain can be measured over time[19]. Studies show that after 1 session using Emotional Freedom Technique (EFT – a Tapping style), results for previously anxious participants were near to normal and were more durable than the results from the comparison group who received Cognitive Behavioral Therapy (CBT). The CBT participants required more sessions to achieve the same results and the results were not as enduring.

In other studies[20], results showed that the stress levels of participants remained well below the levels they tested at prior to the workshop. When tested again months later, their stress results were still lower than when first tested. Something had fundamentally changed within the way they responded to their regular every day stressors.

Balancing the body's energy system

The tapping points come directly from meridians, the Chinese system of energy channels which were mapped out over 5,000 years ago. With my background in traditional Chinese medicine, using the meridian points to create change made sense to me. I felt comfortable tapping on the points instead of using needles since acupressure is a recognised variant of acupuncture. I was a TCM practitioner, but you don't need to become a doctor of traditional

Chinese medicine to use Tapping effectively. You just need to use the techniques frequently and systematically. Your proof will be in your results.

Tapping, like TCM, addresses the entire mind-body system and doesn't distinguish between the mind and the body the way western medicine does. To be healthy in both body and mind, our energy system must be balanced. According to TCM, negative stress, and other unwanted emotions, disrupt the correct movement of this energy, which has a knock on effect on our physical and emotional state. This can be illustrated within a western medicine framework as well as we are now aware that our emotions can contribute to illness. Tapping allows us to remove disruptions (unhelpful beliefs), restore correct movement (appropriate chemical /emotional response) and continue on our path to wellbeing.

As mentioned above, along the meridians are acupuncture or acupressure points. These points provide access to the entire physical and energetic system of the human body. When a needle, pressure or tapping stimulates a point, it has an influence over the mind-body system as a whole.

The tapping process creates change by influencing the way energy flows around the system. When I was still using needles in my acupuncture practice, I would explain that the needles acted like a valve. If there's too much or too little energy at a particular point, the needle acts as a conduit to release or encourage energy and thus restore the balance and flow of energy around the body.

Whilst more research is required, galvanic skin testing[21] (measuring the relative positive or negative charge at any point) reports that there are some differences in the charge on the skin at acupuncture points, indicating more or less energy. There are questions around the ability of current technology to accurately measure these differences and replicate results making the accurate assessment of the influence of an acupuncture needle problematic. In my mind, a fluctuating charge at specific points illustrates the idea that the body is a complex electrical system and that there are ways it can be influenced. By stimulating the point we are drawing attention to an imbalance and the body addresses it – thus restoring balance and wellbeing.

Imaginary Tapping

'Imaginary Tapping' is a more advanced skill where, instead of physically tapping, we simply imagine tapping on the points whilst following the sequence and yes – still experience change. (This is extremely valuable skill when to physically tap would make you look slightly deranged!)

If we're not actually physically influencing a specific point, how do we achieve results? The answer lies in the teachings of NLP. Remember that the brain doesn't know what's real and what's not. The brain reacts to what we 'feel' about a thing/experience to decide what to do. The brain reacts to the meaning we give things. You know this because you can make yourself stressed just by thinking of something that upsets you even though it is not actually occurring. Therefore, thinking about tapping on the points gives your brain the same input as actually doing it. Imaginary Tapping can take more practice. To begin with I do recommend actually physically tapping.

Biofeedback

Biofeedback[22] is also a well-documented technique that can be used to influence the stress response. Biofeedback uses guided imagery, breathing and mindfulness amongst other things to decrease the stress response. This can be monitored and recorded. (FasterEFT uses versions of these techniques; paying attention to your breathing, visualising your stress and observing the changes).

Given our understanding of biofeedback, we know we are able to powerfully influence our health and wellbeing just by thinking about the thing that we want to change, gauging our level of upset, implementing the tapping protocol (either physically or mentally), gauging our level of success and repeating the process.

Which technique is for me?

There are various techniques used within the practices of EFT and FasterEFT. I have shown you one of the tools of the FasterEFT style and there are many more. There are also many differences between the two styles, with the actual tapping itself being the common element. I used EFT for many years and now use FasterEFT. In my experience it creates faster results. Below is an illustration of the FasterEFT points.

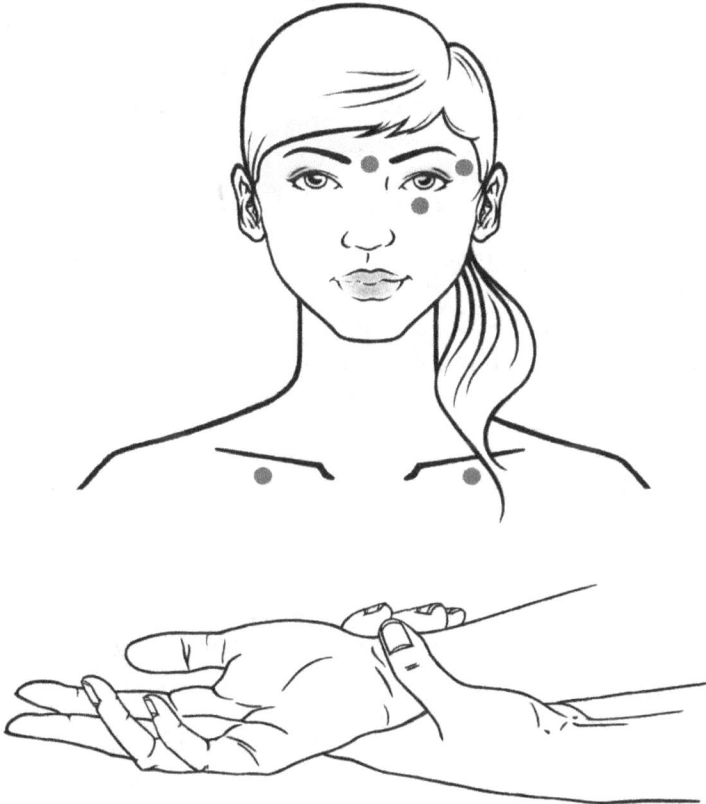

We use these points because they are accessible to practitioners and clients, they cover most of the 12 meridians and the number and location of points is easy to remember. (With FasterEFT we use fewer points than with EFT. Results are achievable regardless of which system of points you choose to incorporate into your personal tapping practice.)

Below you will find an abridged description of the major organ associated with the meridian point and the major emotion associated with the organ.

Eyebrow point (Bladder 2) – Predominately deals with trauma.

Temple (Gall Bladder 4) – Predominately deals with internal conflict. Most tappers use a slightly different location called the 'side of the eye' point or Gall Bladder 1. I use Gall Bladder 4 at the temple because it's on the same meridian and is out of the way for clients who wear glasses.

Under the Eye (Stomach 2) – Predominately deals with anxiety.

Collar bone (Kidney 27) – Predominately deals with fear.

Squeezing the Wrist – Covers Lung (grief), Large Intestine (letting go), Pericardium (emotional emptiness), Heart (hysteria/shock), Triple Burner (despair) and Small Intestine (fear of change).

Naming the meridians with terms from western medicine doesn't mean there's a direct relationship with the organ of the same name (as described by western medicine). Remember, we are working with an understanding of anatomy from 5000 years ago. Consider these 'organs' as 'personalities' with particular strengths and weakness. Most importantly, each 'personality' has a specific emotion associated with it.

If you find yourself gravitating towards a specific point or two, as many of my clients have done, try looking up the emotion associated with that particular 'personality'. My experienced clients often find they get big shifts in their emotions when they get to certain points. I have come to call these points, which vary from client to client, 'power points'. In almost all cases, when we look at the corresponding emotions associated with the meridian and 'personality' associated with their 'power point', they are exactly the emotions the client is working with the most.

The mystery of the mind-body connection is glorious and intriguing. I hope I can inspire you to honour your mind and your body. If you'd like to investigate TCM for more inspiring insights, see the resources section for some good references[23].

What can I expect to feel?

Many of my clients ask me what they will feel during the tapping process. Some are already emotionally stretched to the limit and get concerned that they'll go into some overwhelming reaction that they may be unable to cope with. Emotions do come up, and that's the point. Then we get to deal with them. I reassure them they will never leave feeling worse than when they walked in. If they are focused and disciplined during the process and do not settle until they are below a 2 out of 10, they may never feel the same way again about that emotion or experience. They'll feel transformed in a very real way.

My goal is that they can no longer find the resources they'd been using, up to that point, to maintain their problem. When we can no longer find the resources that keep a problem in place, we cannot have a problem. The mind cannot react to something it can no longer access. You can dismantle the rules of the game that you have operated from for your whole life up to this point by transforming the emotions that make those rules 'so'. If you dismantle an emotion, you are also dismantling the beliefs around it.

What's so exciting to many of my clients, (and still to me even after all of these years), is that Tapping and the other techniques that formulate the FasterEFT model, dismantle emotions by using feelings and the senses. Feelings like the sensations – tightness, sharpness, heaviness, sounds, tastes, memories, pictures, the 'how you know' – we use these things to dismantle the emotions and change the rules of our game.

Typically, my clients find the feelings morph, change, move and decrease over the course of their session. If I'm doing my job properly, by the end of the session they can no longer find their problem or the feelings associated with it even if I ask them to bring it back. If they can bring the problem back I ask them, 'How did you do that?' Perhaps they remembered something that was said and that bought the feeling back, perhaps they saw a picture in their mind and that bought it back, perhaps they remembered a smell from that time and that bought it back. Once we know 'how' the problem can be bought back we can use that information to understand the dominant resources the client tends to use. We then dismantle the resource by changing it or removing it during the next round of tapping then test again. Of course, you can reintroduce experiences and re-educate the body and mind to stress again if you wish to. I encourage all of my clients to actively test their results out in the real world as well. What's consistently reported back to me is that they simply cannot get as stressed about the same negative experiences or that it takes a great deal more of the negative stimulation for them to feel triggered in any way.

By the end of the session clients walk out feeling relaxed, surprised, elated and just plain different. And you can too.

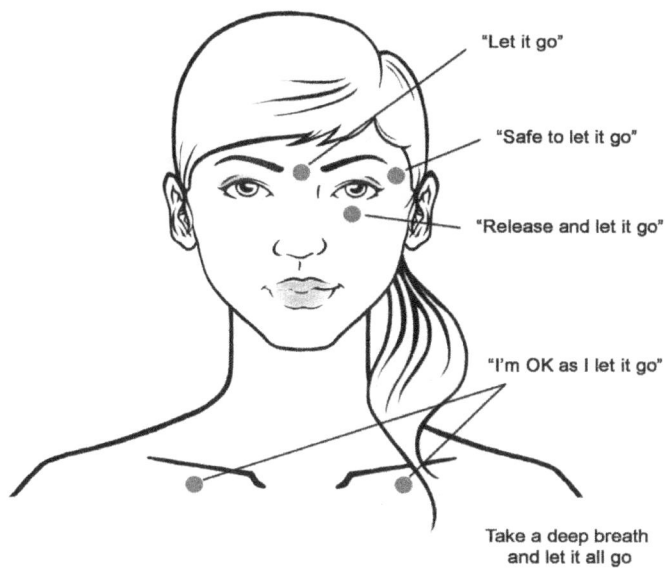

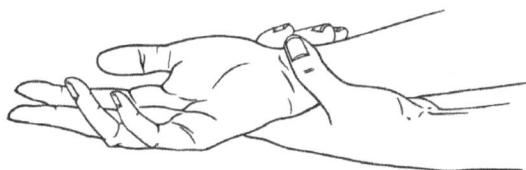

"Let it go"

"Safe to let it go"

"Release and let it go"

"I'm OK as I let it go"

Take a deep breath
and let it all go

Say:
"Peace"

www.drlindawilson.com

Summary

- Whilst the mechanism of change through Tapping remains unclear, the results are measurable and verifiable.

- FasterEFT uses elements of TCM, NLP, hypnosis, mindfulness, physical touch and an understanding of the way the mind processes and gets results.

- We create balance in the mind and body when we use Tapping.

- There are different styles of Tapping.

- When Tapping is used correctly your stress will be transformed.

NOTES

NOTES

Chapter 16

5 Keys for ADAPTability

I want to introduce my ADAPTability model to you now so that you are aware not only of 'what' to do but the processing sequence behind it. You deserve an inside peek!

I became aware that I operate in a predictable and consistent way when I am with my clients. It begins from the time the client walks through the door. The methodology is just as powerful for my clients whether they are a stressed out lawyer on the verge of a meltdown, a 6-year-old bed wetter or an 86-year-old insomniac. I teach my clients this same step-by-step methodology so they get maximum results. This means when they leave the calm safe haven of my room and go out in to their real world, they have the tools and techniques required to take care of themselves and an understanding of where they are up to in the process. I have come to refer to the model as the 5 Keys for ADAPTability.

The Keys are a step through looping process. The process has been very specifically named ADAPTability because *adaptation* has enabled the survival of our species and an *ability* is a skill that improves with practice. Life throws us curve balls and we learn, adapt, learn and adapt again as we grow – often without consciously questioning the rules about life. We adapt physically and emotionally and most of the time we do so unconsciously. Even though we have little control over unforeseen and unexpected events, we do have the ability to adapt to circumstances and situations. We do this millions of times as we learn about the world and how to stay safe and happy in it.

Unfortunately, the older we become the more resistant we can be to the concept of adaptability. It takes on negative connotations as though we're 'giving in' or sacrificing something. My definition of being able to adapt is accepting there is *difference* out there in our world and that we're able to not just cope with it but also learn incredible things from it. Some of the differences we cope with without a second thought. They are familiar enough not to create a need for adaptation of our thinking or feeling. Some differences we are unable to adapt to without internal struggle that can include a lot of emotional pain and stress. Stress is one of the many outcomes we experience when confronted with differences.

Often subtle differences over time can generate significant stress but we may be unable to put our finger on why we just feel 'wrong'. The loving partner who slowly turns into a control freak can create enormous confusion as the rules of the game change in ways that are difficult to verbalise. We adapt to these subtle stresses largely unconsciously until something significant makes us truly uncomfortable.

I want to bring ADAPTability into your conscious awareness. I want you to feel you have control over yourself, even when life feels out of control. I want you to be able to use your newfound abilities to help you to adapt in the way best for *you*. Using ADAPTability, I see you being able to consciously adapt when life deals up the unexpected with the result being your emotions and physical health staying in really good shape even though you might go through some really tough stuff.

I believe that if we're able to positively adapt in ways that are good for us and those around us, nothing can happen that we cannot reshape or reframe. With ADAPTability we get to choose our responses and feelings to those events. With the increase in health challenges we face as individuals and as a global community, having ADAPTability is already critical. I hope you choose to develop this skill and teach it to others, especially those who will inherit the legacy of a world faced with innumerable challenges.

So, what are the 5 Keys for ADAPTability and Stress made Easy?

1.   A – Assessment

2.   D – Distillation

3.   A – Association

4.   P – Processing

5.   T – Testing

1 *Assessment* is about identifying the problem.

Sometimes my clients find their struggles very hard to express. Often they are high achievers, aged 35 – 50, who have hit a brick wall and realise they've simply run out of steam. They often feel guilty that they have no energy for their work, partner, kids or friendships. They feel a sense of disappointment that they have reached this stage in their life and it's not a reflection of what they anticipated. Nothing feels as good as they had hoped. Because of these emotions, they're concerned that their relationships, work or other commitments are at risk in some way as they struggle to have them *mean* anything. It's often at this time that my clients have affairs, get divorced, have another baby, have a breakdown or engage in other types of risky behaviors to try to shake something up.

Disappointment, confusion and disconnection mean these clients have a deep fear of being exposed as having *failed*. This is a deeply personal and painful realisation that takes great courage to face even though the surface reality may be far from reflecting failure.

Whilst you might not be fully aware of what is generating your stress, the great news is that if you can identify through your senses what your body is physically experiencing when you have these emotions, then you can make incredible changes in very short periods of time.

2 *Distillation* means choosing one issue to focus on.

We are often so overwhelmed by our emotions that everything just becomes a great big messy clump. The distillation process creates clarity. Clarity ensures a focused impact on your stress and enables excellent results as each clarification is achieved and tested.

3 *Associating* to the problem by getting 'in' your stressed state and scoring it 0–10.

Getting specific about what you're experiencing or feeling when you're 'in' your stressed state provides you with all the information you need to proceed. This association can come through any of the senses. Numbness is a feeling, as is tightness in the chest. You might hear sounds, feel physical or emotional pain, anger, sadness etc. With lots of safeguards in place I ask my clients to 'feel it as if it were happening right now'. I ask them to pay attention to what they can feel in their body as they think about the problem. The more these feelings can be associated with, the faster they are transformed when we move to the next step.

4 *Processing*. Start to implement the tapping technique of FasterEFT.

Using the FasterEFT Quick Tap protocol means you address both the mind's perceptions (as you have activated the mind by focusing on the problem), and the body's reactions (by recognising how the body has reacted to your thoughts). This process is easy to learn and allows you to be the director of your emotions and feelings rather than being victim to them.

5 *Testing* by going back to the problem to reassess your score.

This step is vital. With this testing process you will immediately be able to assess the level of change. You'll have all the evidence you need to feel encouraged to continue and refine the process for yourself. When you're feeling overwhelmed, stressed or vulnerable this is especially important.

After you test your results you loop back to step 1 and continue to work with the same problem or, once resolved, decide what to focus on next.

Once you are familiar with this information you might recognise that the Quick Tap process is a mini ADAPTability model: Assess (choose your problem), Distill (get very specific by going to the feeling), Associate (focus on the feeling and score it), Process (start to tap), Test (check your score).

NOTES

NOTES

Chapter 17

Change right here right now and become your own favourite person

Here we are at the culmination of the book and I trust it's helped you make, at the very least, some small breakthroughs and brought you some stress relief. I hope you now understand that you can be the creator in your own game and not just a player in it.

I hope you have learnt that being aware of, catching and directing your thinking can change everything and that this requires being fully present. As we have discussed, many of us spend the majority of our lives either in the past, or in the future and rarely in the present. This means we are rarely right here, right now. But, right here, right now is the only moment we have any influence or power. Right here, right now is where relationships happen, including the one with ourselves. My guess is you yearn for the authentic connections we can only feel when we are really present to those around us, and especially when we are present to ourselves.

By learning and applying the strategies in this book, you will become your favourite person to be with and the mastermind of your mind.

If you spend time determining that *who you are* is really *who you want to be* by taking a look at the problems in your life, you might discover so much more about yourself than you ever imagined. If you don't already, learn to enjoy your own company. You are already successfully producing what you hold within you. If you don't like it, use the techniques, use them often and change it. See what you find out about yourself and I hope you get to LOVE spending time with you, relaxed, content, in control.

Change your mind, change your health

By following the advice in this book, you are choosing to literally 'change your mind' so it can become a powerful, unique and fun place to be. If we are going to spend so much time using our mind (a lifetime to be exact), we should at least be running the show and having some fun. And guess what? You now know it is simple. Just ONE better question and one straight forward technique and your mind is yours to cherish, respect and use to achieve the peaceful states that enable you to be the best version of yourself, compassionate, powerful, resilient and creative. Choose YOU.

If at any point you feel like you're not getting anywhere, read through the chapter summaries I have recapped below, and remind yourself that you are not broken and that each and every thought is potentially a new beginning.

Chapter 1: Why do we feel stress? – Because we can

Summary
- We are just as capable of being happy as we are of being stressed.
- Stress is a lazy response because it doesn't require consciousness and evaluation.
- Happiness requires an active choice.

- Remaining curious about our reactions can help us change them.
- The good news is you can get to choose.

Chapter 2: The game of life is set up with inherited rules – but you can change them

Summary

- There are rules to our game of life.
- We learn them before we are consciously aware we are doing so.
- We apply them, most of the time, without being consciously aware we are doing so.
- If we are lucky they work, if not we feel everyone else is cheating at the game.
- As we grow we have the potential to assess our rules and decide, 'Are these the rules I want to live by?'

Chapter 3: A simple example of 'The Set Up' – the complex weaving of ourselves

Summary

- Rules of life are inherited from those who raise us.
- There are infinite variations in the rules.
- Whilst life may be unpredictable, the way we react to things is always according to our rules.
- Most of the time we don't know how to get new rules, even if we know we need them. We ask 'Why?'
- Sometimes, we find a way to rewrite our rulebook by asking better questions like, When, Who, Where, What, and How.

Chapter 4: There are no broken people – we're just playing with outdated rules

Summary

- You're not broken, you're just operating from a set of rules that no longer serve you.

- You can manage stress by addressing the meaning you apply to the stressor (trigger) and changing it if required.

- You cannot change anyone else; they have to do that for themselves.

- When you change what's within you the whole world and everyone in it looks different.

- The more you identify your 'meaning making', the easier it gets to change it.

Chapter 5: Meaning makes the difference – to you and me and everyone around us

Summary

- Stress impacts every system within the body – especially if we believe it will.

- More and more research is discovering that what we think directly impacts our body, down to the gene level.

- What happens in the mind also happens in the body.

- You can use the body to address the mind and the mind to address the body.

- If you don't address both the mind and the body simultaneously results are muted.

Chapter 6: You – a hamster on the wheel of repeating rules

Summary

- We repeat behaviours even when we want to stop because we haven't changed our internal environment, rules and expectations.

- Even the best will in the world won't be strong enough to maintain a decision to change if the change we hope for is too different to what we have going on inside of us in the rules department.

- There are lots of reasons we do what we do but they always come down to what we hold within us. Most of the time we hold onto the rules we know because they are to do with 'belonging' and 'placement'.

- We can feel helpless to change.

- Change is possible.

Chapter 7: Having unrealistic expectations – a war with reality

Summary

- We bring our perceptions and beliefs to every situation, even when they're wrong.

- Numbness is also a feeling usually generated by overwhelm.

- Your feelings, or lack there of, are an opportunity.

- Asking the 'Why?' question keeps us in a victim state.

- Persist – this means you might fail. Persist anyway, just start with the strongest feeling.

Chapter 8: What happens in the brain when we're stressed? – Chemical meaning making

Summary

- Your brain and body are connected chemically and through 'experience'.

- Your level of stress and your interpretation of that stress in any given moment can determine whether you are a creative genius or a violent offender.

- When we understand the way our brain operates we can create solutions using exactly the same 'hardware' and 'software' that interprets our experiences.

- Working with the natural flow of the mind is the best way to create fast change.

- You can use your body to influence and understand your mind.

Chapter 9: Resource States. Asking better questions to get better answers – the only way forward

Summary

- Going after different results in your life can take courage.

- You may feel very uncomfortable along the way as you are challenged to adapt.

- Learning to ask better questions makes all the difference.

- Asking better questions makes you the creator of your game not just a player in it.

- Asking better questions enables adaptability.

Chapter 10: Two Models of the World – you get to choose; above or below

Summary

- We can live below or above the line, but it is our choice and our choice alone.

- We can directly influence our emotions using our feelings to move us above the line or to keep us below the line.

- There are benefits to living below the line – we get to be victims and it can never be our fault. We also get to continue our addictions. This way of living is self-perpetuating. We allow our emotions and feelings to perpetuate our way of being.

- The most powerful difference between 'above' and 'below' is the questions we ask.

- There are benefits to living above the line – we get to be solution finders and leaders. We also get to do a lot of the things we love because we know that doing so sustains us. This way of living is self-perpetuating. We use our feelings to manipulate our negative emotions.

Chapter 11: The Ultimate POWER Question – When you get stuck, ask yourself, 'How do I know I have this problem?'

Summary

- The only way we really know we have a problem is because we feel it.

- When we go 'looking' for a feeling we reconnect our mind with our body.

- We have no chance of helping others resolve their problems unless they're ready.

- Heal yourself first and then what you bring to the world is a healer.

- Deal with yourself first and then teach others by example.

Chapter 12: The faster we become aware the faster we can repair

Summary

- The faster we become aware the faster we can repair.

- We gain power by bringing awareness and focus to our feelings and emotions.

- Step back far enough and you can become the non-judgmental observer of your emotions.

- Noticing what is happening within us takes practice.

- Our body is our greatest ally.

NOTES

NOTES

Afterword

I dream of a future where holistic healthcare becomes the norm; where integrative wellness is the way we deal with emotional problems such as stress, depression and anxiety or indeed any other mental health issue. We can't continue to be a culture obsessed with and force-fed negativity. We must make the much more conscious choice to surround ourselves with positive influences, mindfulness and self-awareness by creating and reflecting on the wonders and joys of life; by revisiting as often as possible those moments that fill us with love and optimism, focus and energy.

We can't continue to be a drug culture. It's expensive, creates dependence, is non sustainable and does not deal with the causes of disease, only the symptoms. The tools in Stress Made Easy create independence not dependence.

Peel yourself off the ceiling over and over before you reach that point where you're unable to catch yourself. You can take responsibility for your internal world.

If you are a professional researcher and you're intrigued, curious, skeptical or even dismissive of these techniques, prove to me (and the thousands of individuals who successfully use these techniques), that my experiences and the results of my clients are wrong. I challenge you.

On the other hand and with a bit of a positive reframe, if you are a researcher out there who is intrigued, curious, skeptical or even dismissive of these techniques, I invite you to be educated and experience the difference these techniques make. Familiarise yourself with the work of Dawson Church and Professor Tony Stewart[24], (who has helped introduced EFT to the National Health Service in the UK). Sample some of the hundreds of client session videos of Robert G. Smith or the thousands of anecdotal testimonials from his clients worldwide. Book in for a session – you might become one of Tapping's greatest proponents!

The fact is, we can't afford to ignore potential solutions when we are failing using the current system. My feeling is that things should be assumed helpful until they are shown not to be, not the other way around. Traditional Chinese Medicine (TCM) was dismissed until western medical science had evolved enough to have the appropriate tools to measure it's efficacy. Now you see TCM integrated into large mainstream institutions. Dr's of TCM work alongside mainstream western medicine practitioners with GP's getting trained themselves so that they can offer it to patients. Awesome – now let's keep moving forward with the leading edge tools of Tapping and achieve even more.

Although this is the Afterword of the book, the final words will not be mine they will be yours. I leave you in the hope that you will continue to write chapters in your own life, on purpose. I hope you will revisit old scripts and rewrite them to suit your life as it is now and as you want it to be.

You deserve the life you dream of and now you can create it, consciously, authentically and on purpose. I wish you the very, very best of new beginnings.

NOTES

NOTES

Selected resources, references and recommended reading

Chapter 1

1. Safe Work Australia (2013, April). *Incidence of Accepted Workers Compensation Claims for Mental Stress in Australia.* Retrieved on 25/3/14 from http://safeworkaustralia.gov.au/sites/swa/about/publications/pages/workers-compensation-claims-for-mental-stress-in-australia

2. Work Safe Australia health and safety topics published 2011. Retrieved on 25/3/14 from http://www.worksafe.vic.gov.au/safety-and-prevention/health-and-safety-topics/stress

Chapter 4

3. Robert G Smith, Founder of Faster Emotionally Focused Transformations (FasterEFT). http://www.fastereft.com

Chapter 5

4. Keller, A., Litzelman. K., Wisk, L. E., Maddox, T., Cheng, E. R., Creswell, P. D., Witt, W. P. (2012 Sep). Does the perception that stress affects health matter? The association with health and mortality. *Health Psychology*, 31(5):677–84. doi: 10.1037/a0026743.

5. Jamieson, J. P., Nock, M. K., Department of Psychology, Harvard University; Mendes, W. B., Department of Psychiatry, University of California San Francisco. (2012). Improving

Acute Stress Responses: The Power of Reappraisal. *Journal of Experimental Psychology*, General, Vol 141(3), 417–422. doi: 10.1037/a0025719.

6. McGonigal, K. (2013, June). Kelly McGonigal: How to make stress your friend [Video file]. Retrieved on 25/3/14 from http://youtu.be/RcGyVTAoXEU.

7. Goetzel, R. Z., Anderson et. al. (1998, Oct) *American Journal of Occupational and Environmental Medicine*, 40; 10. October 1998; 843–854.

8. This figure is quoted by Smith, F. Stress (2013, Sep): Stress: the new workplace epidemic. *The Australian Financial Review*. Retrieved on 25/3/14 from http://www. afr.com/p/national/stress_the_new_workplace_epidemic_ E5MDtPWbXsVuIgxil07CiN

9. The ACE (Adverse Childhood Experiences) Study. Centers for Disease Control and Prevention and Kaiser Permanente's Health Appraisal Clinic in San Diego. For further information visit http://acestudy.org

10. The top 10 killers of adults correlated with unhealed emotional wounds included cancer, heart disease, diabetes, high blood pressure, obesity, hepatitis, sexually transmitted diseases. Smoking, intravenous drug abuse, depression, unintended pregnancy and suicide attempts also correlated with higher ACE scores. Retrieved on 25/3/14 from http://acestudy.org

11. Rein, G., Atkinson. M., & McCraty, R. (1995). The Physiological and Psychological Effects of Compassion and Anger. *Journal of Advancement in Medicine*, 8(2):87–105. Retrieved on 25/3/14 from HeartMath Institute website, http:// www.heartmath.org/free-services/solutions-for-stress/solutions-immune-system.html

12. Dr Pert, C. (2010). *Molecules of Emotion*. NY: Scribner.

13. Church, D. (2009). *Genie in your Genes*. CA: Energy Psychology Press.

Chapter 8

14. To discover more about what happens in the brain when we're stressed see:

    The website of The Franklin Institute Resources for Science Learning http://www.fi.edu/learn/brain/stress.html#how

    Also, an informative YouTube video presentation by Dr John Kenworthy, http://www.youtube.com/watch?v=gmwiJ6ghLIM

Chapter 13

15. Jewell, K. (2013). *From Stress to Success: The Secrets to Fast, Permanent Life Change with FasterEFT*. US: CreateSpace.

16. Wilson, L. (Presenter). 2014. Introduction to The Quick Tap. [Video file]. Retrieved on 25/3/14 from http://www.drlindawilson.com

17. **Australian Tapping Practitioners**

    Victoria

    Sarah Batsanis – *Reservoir*
    0424 128 020
    www.fastereft.com.au

    Keith Hulstaert – *Burwood*
    0409 546 549
    www.sectretpath.com.au

Helen O'Connor – *Preston*
(03) 9484 7276
www.helenoconnor.com.au

Heather Wilks – *Carnegie*
0414 836 652
www.ohnaturale.com

Pam Wright – *Geelong*
Pam Wright and Associates
1800 814 313
www.pamwright.com.au

Canberra – Australian Capital Territory

Deirdre Brocklebank
0412 605 274

Overseas Tapping Researchers and/or Practitioners
Emotional Freedom Techniques
Dawson Church USA
Gary Craig USA
Nick Ortner USA
Professor Tony Stewart UK
Dr Peta Stapleton AUST

Faster Emotionally Focused Transformations

FasterEFT
Robert G Smith USA
www.fastereft.com

Deirdre Maguire IRELAND
www.fastereft.co.uk
www.steppingstonesni.co.uk

Chapter 14

18. Wilson, L. (Presenter). 2014. Dissecting The Quick Tap. [Video file]. Retrieved on 25/3/14 from http://www.drlindawilson.com

Chapter 15 – How tapping works

19. This research study can be found on the website of Innersource: The Neurological Foundations of Energy Psychology – Brain Scan Changes During 4 Weeks of Treatment for Generalized Anxiety Disorder – 12 Sessions Combining Manual Acupoint Stimulation and Image Activation. Retrieved 25/3/14 from http://www.innersource. net/ep/articlespublished/neurological-foundations.html

Church, D., Hawk, C., Brooks, A., Toukolehto, O., Wren, M., Dinter, I., & Stein, P. (2013). Psychological trauma in veterans using EFT (Emotional Freedom Techniques): A randomized controlled trial. *Journal of Nervous and Mental Disease*, 201, 153–160. doi: 10.1097/NMD.0b013e31827f6351.

Karatzias, T., Power, K., Brown, K., McGoldrick, T., Begum, M., Young, J., … & Adams, S. (2011). A controlled comparison of the effectiveness and efficiency of two psychological therapies for posttraumatic stress disorder: eye movement desensitization and reprocessing vs. emotional freedom techniques. *Journal of Nervous and Mental Disease*, 199(6), 372–378.

Church, D., & Brooks, A. J. (2012). CAM and Energy Psychology Techniques Remediate PTSD Symptoms in Veterans and Spouses. Paper presented at the Association for Comprehensive

Energy Psychology conference, San Diego, June 5, 2012. Submitted for publication.

20. Church, D., Yount, G., & Brooks, A. J. (2012). The effect of Emotional Freedom Techniques (EFT) on stress biochemistry: A randomized controlled trial. *Journal of Nervous and Mental Disease*, 200(10), 891–896. doi: 10.1097/NMD.0b013e31826b9fc1.

   Church, D., & Brooks, A. J. (2010). The effect of a brief EFT (Emotional Freedom Techniques) self-intervention on anxiety, depression, pain and cravings in healthcare workers. *Integrative Medicine: A Clinician's Journal*, 6, 40–44.

   Palmer-Hoffman, J., & Brooks, A. J. (2011). Psychological symptom change after group application of Emotional Freedom Techniques (EFT). *Energy Psychology: Theory, Research, & Treatment*, 3(1), 57–72.

   Rowe, J. E. (2005). The effects of EFT on long-term psychological symptoms. *Counseling and Clinical Psychology*, 2(3), 104–111.

   Retrieved 25/3/14 http://www.innersource.net/ep/images/stories/downloads/Acupoint_Stimulation_Research_Review.pdf

21. Kramer, S., Winterhalter, K., Schober, G., Becker, U., Wiegele, B., Kutz, D. F., Kolb, F. P., Zaps, D., Lang, P. M., Irnich, D. (2009). Characteristics of electrical skin resistance at acupuncture points in healthy humans. *J Altern Complement Medicine*. Retrieved 25/3/14 from http://www.ncbi.nlm.nih.gov/pubmed/19422323

22. Angele McGrady (1994). Effects of group relaxation training and thermal biogreedback on blood pressure and related physiological and psychological variables in essential hypertension. *Biofeedback and Self-regulation Journal*, Volume 19, 1, 51–66. Retrieved 25/3/14 http://link.springer.com/article/10.1007/BF01720670#page-1

23. Beinfield, H, Korngold, E. (1991). *Between Heaven and Earth: A Guide to Chinese Medicine*. NY: Ballantine Books.

   Kaptchuk, T. (2000). *The Web That Has No Weaver: Understanding Chinese Medicine*. NY: McGraw-Hill.

24. Professor Tony Stewart, Clinical Hypnotherapist, EFT Advanced Practitioner and Trainer, Matrix Reimprinting Practitioner and Trainer (UK). Prof Tony Stewart is a Professor in Public Health, a published author and winner of the prestigious BMA award in 2011.

   Prof Stewart and colleagues have been involved in primary EFT research involving students of Staffordshire University and NHS patients. (The National Health Service provides free healthcare for all UK citizens, funded by taxes.)

   For more information on Prof Tony Stewart and his clinical studies see:

   Stewart, A., Boath, E., Carryer, A., Walton, I., Hill, L. (2013). Can Emotional Freedom Techniques (EFT) be effective in the treatment of emotional conditions? Results of a service evaluation in Sandwell. *Journal of Psychological Therapies in Primary Care*, 2013; 2:71–84. Retrieved 25/3/2014 http://www.eft-therapy.org/publications.html

www.ingramcontent.com/pod-product-compliance
Lightning Source LLC
Chambersburg PA
CBHW072134020426
42334CB00018B/1792